Dermatopathology Primer of INFLAMMATORY DISEASES

Steven R. Feldman, MD, PhD

Omar P. Sangueza, MD

Rita Pichardo-Geisinger, MD

Megan A. Kinney, MD, MPH

Ashley Feneran, BS

Swetha Narahari, BS

Department of Dermatology
Wake Forest School of Medicine
Winston-Salem, North Carolina

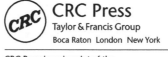

CRC Press
Taylor & Francis Group
Boca Raton London New York

CRC Press is an imprint of the
Taylor & Francis Group, an **informa** business

CRC Press
Taylor & Francis Group
6000 Broken Sound Parkway NW, Suite 300
Boca Raton, FL 33487-2742

© 2014 by Taylor & Francis Group, LLC
CRC Press is an imprint of Taylor & Francis Group, an Informa business

No claim to original U.S. Government works

Printed on acid-free paper
Version Date: 20131023

International Standard Book Number-13: 978-1-4822-2504-4 (Paperback)

Visit the Taylor & Francis Web site at
http://www.taylorandfrancis.com

and the CRC Press Web site at
http://www.crcpress.com

FOREWORD

The task of organizing and developing this book required the creativity of many individuals. We are sincerely grateful to James and Gloria Graham, who donated their personal clinical images and dermatopathology slides to the Wake Forest University library from which many of the photos in this book were taken. The task of digitizing the Graham library required much work, and we would like to thank Will Willner, Vishal Khanna, and Nancy (Liz) Jackman for their contributions.

We would like to thank the Department of Pathology at Wake Forest University and are grateful for their photo contributions.

We would also like to thank our colleagues and residents in the Departments of Dermatology and Pathology for their honest input in the creation of this book. We especially thank the residents who took time from their busy schedules to give their opinions on both the book and on the subject of dermatopathology.

INTRODUCTION

When discussing the subject of dermatopathology with a second year resident, he said, "It's like a brick wall that you keep hitting—over and over again". Eventually you break through that initial barrier and get a grasp of the material, but it might not even be until the second year of residency until you begin to do so.

It would be difficult to try and memorize 2,000 histopathological findings for different skin diseases by categorizing them in your mind as distinct, separate entities. Using the pathologic basis provides one way to categorize the diseases, but this approach does not lend itself to converting histological characteristics to the diagnosis. Nevertheless, this was the standard approach to dermatopathology not long ago. Instead, an ordered, structured approach based on histology characteristics presents an ideal means of organizing our understanding of dermatopathology and more easily coming to a diagnosis based on the histological findings. Once the basic structure of this organizational scheme is understood—something that can be quickly grasped by new residents in dermatology and pathology—more detailed, complex and rarer conditions can be understood within a greater hierarchy of subjects. Thus, one begins with the understanding of the skeletal structure, then adding on more flesh as one delves deeper into dermatopathology.

The intent of this book is to introduce the new resident to dermatopathology in an easily approachable format that can be reviewed in the first month (ideally the first few days) of their training. This guide is a general overview to be used to refresh the learner on general principles of histopathology and to establish an outline of the subject. Each topic is illustrated within a flow chart showing similar diseases by histology and where it lies in the greater scheme of dermatopathology. In this format, we hope for residents to be less intimidated by the vastness and intricacies of the subject. We present a basic design that can be easily added to as residents learn the subject in greater detail throughout their training. Perhaps in this way dermatopathology will not resemble such a 'brick wall' and can be understood much earlier to help complement the rest of their dermatology studies.

CONTRIBUTORS

AUTHOR	SECTIONS
Ali Alikhan, MD	Pityriasis lichenoides, Pityriasis rosea, Seborrheic dermatitis, Dermatophytosis, Polyarteritis nodosa, Leprosy, Sarcoidosis, Granuloma faciale, Pemphigus vulgaris
Jennifer Ang, MD	Cryoglobulinemia
Elizabeth Bailey MD, MPH	Cryptococcosis
Joshua Black, MD	Graft versus host disease
Patrick Blake, MD	Tuberculosis, Sporotrichosis
Ranti Bolaji, MD	Herpes simplex virus
Renata Brindise, DO	Androgenetic alopecia, Alopecia areata
Tracy Burns, BS	Pemphigus vulgaris, Pityriasis rubra pilaris
Daniel Bryan, PA-C, MPAS, BS	Granuloma annulare, Aspergillosis
Rebecca Chain	Blastomycosis, Coccidiodomycosis
Jennifer Channual	Necrobiosis lipoidica
Lily Cheng, BS	Granuloma faciale
Jacqueline DeLuca, MD	Dermatomyositis
Meghan Dubina, MD	Grover's disease
Samira Farouk, BS	Mucormycosis
Ashley Feneran, BS	Pigmented purpuric dermatitis, Tinea versicolor, Central centrifugal scarring alopecia
Michael Ghods	Lichen nitidus, Pityriasis lichenoides, Leprosy
Jamie Goldberg, MD	Lichen Planus
Elizabeth Heaton, BA	Small vessel leukocytoclastic vasculitis
Abraar Karan, BA	Dermatophytosis
Ravneet Kaur BSN, MD	Polymorphous light eruption, Miliaria

Elizabeth Kiracofe, BS	**Urticaria, Erythema multiforme, Arthropod bites, Dermatitis herpetiformis**
Smitha Kuppalli, MD	Stasis dermatitis
Katrina Lam	**Lichen simplex chronicus**
Patricia Li	Sarcoidosis
Swetha Narahari, BS	**Subacute and chronic spongiotic dermatitis, Reactions to foreign materials, Staphlococcal scalded skin Syndrome**
Kelly K. Park, MD	Sweet's syndrome, Erythema elevatum diutinum, Pyoderma gangrenosum
Catherine M. Pham, MD	**Erythema annulare centrifugum**
Grace Prince, BS	Molluscum contagiosum
Annahita Sarcon, MS	**Acute spongiotic dermatits, Bullous pemphigoid**
Robin Schroeder, BS	Pitted keratolysis, Scabies, Impetigo
Alyssa Searles, MD	**Porphyria cutanea tarda**
Avnee Shah, MD	Urticaria, Psoriasis, Trichotillomania
Mary Sockolov	**Polyarteritis nodosa, Seborrheic dermatitis, Pityriasis rosea**
Betsy Uhlenhake, MD	Erythema nodosum, Lipodermatosclerosis, Lupus panniculitis, Traumatic fat necrosis, Morphea
Pooja Virmani	**Viral exanthems, Fixed drug eruption**
Nahid Yakuby, BA	Porokeratosis
Lindsay Young, MD	**Cryoglobulinemia**

TABLE OF CONTENTS

SUPERFICIAL PERIVASCULAR DERMATITIS

- ### SUPERFICIAL PERIVASCULAR DERMATITIS

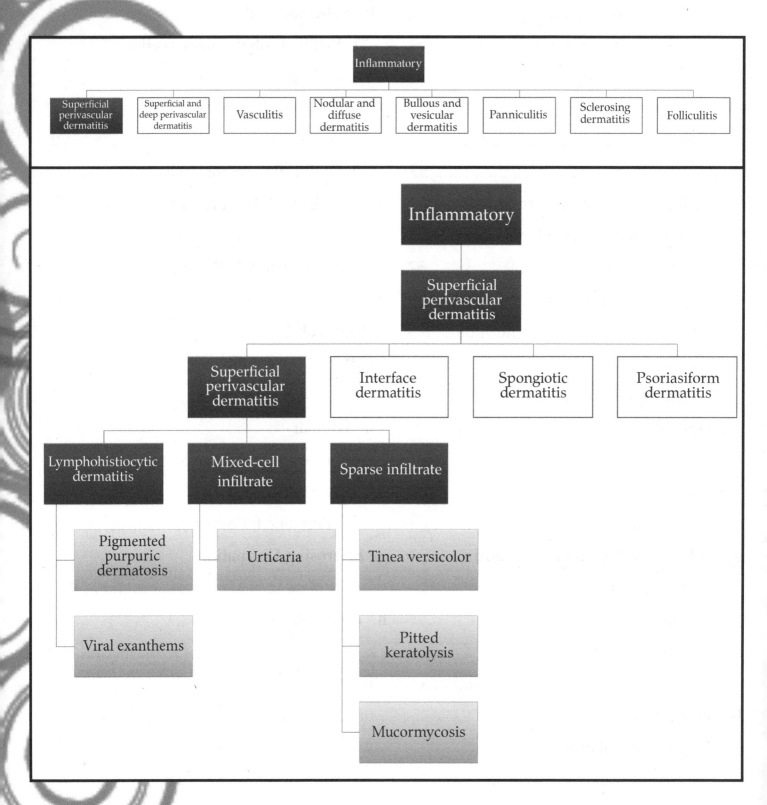

PIGMENTED PURPURIC DERMATOSIS

Pigmented purpuric dermatosis (PPD) is a term that envelops a group of diseases that are similar in clinical and dermatopathologic presentation. They are clinically characterized by petechiae and pigmentation, and histologically by hemosiderin deposits and capillaritis.

HISTOLOGICAL FEATURES

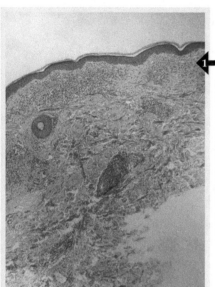

1. Mild perivascular and interstitial lymphohistiocytic infiltrate in papillary dermis

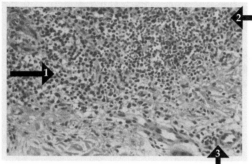

1. **Lymphocytes**
2. **Extravasated erythrocytes**
3. **Capillaritis with perivascular infiltrate**

Other Features:
- Hemosiderin laden macrophages

HISTOLOGICAL DIFFERENTIAL

STATIS DERMATITIS (SD)

- Extends deeper into dermis
- More pronounced epidermal changes
- More fibrosis of dermis

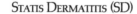

GOOD THINGS TO KNOW

PPD dermatopathology results are nearly identical in all variants. So awareness of the varying clincial presentations will aid in diagnosis.

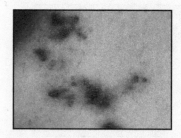

EPIDEMIOLOGY

- Common in females 30–60
- Unknown etiology
- Risk factors:
  - Venous stasis or insufficiency
  - Certain drugs
  - Pressure
  - Trauma

PATHOPHYSIOLOGY

- Results from inflammation and hemorrhage of superficial papillary dermal vessels, typically capillaries

CLINICAL FEATURES

- Usually asymptomatic with minimal pruritis, and lesions usually present as petechiae or patches, not purpura.
- Eruptions favor the lower extremities.
- Lesions range from "cayenne pepper" red to yellow or brown.

SPECIAL STUDIES

- None

CLINICAL VARIANTS

- Schamberg's disease
- Majocchi's disease
- Gougerot–Blum disease
- Itching purpura
- Lichen aureus

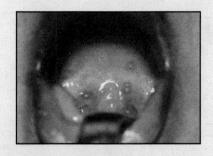

EPIDEMIOLOGY

• Onset usually occurs before 20 years of age.
• Transmitted by inhalation, food, blood, or sexual contact.
• Worldwide distribution.

PATHOPHYSIOLOGY

• Antigen–antibody complex deposition causing inflammation

CLINICAL FEATURES

• Produce a wide variety of generalized mucocutaneous manifestations
• Erythematous maculopapular eruption
• Petechiae
• Conjunctivitis (measles)

SPECIAL STUDIES

• None

CLINICAL VARIANTS

• Roseola infantum (exanthem subitum, sixth disease)
• Erythema infectiosum (fifth disease)
• Rubella (German measles)
• Measles

VIRAL EXANTHEMS

An exanthem is a skin eruption occurring as a symptom of primary systemic disease. Widespread exanthems are a manifestation of some viral infections.

HISTOLOGICAL FEATURES

1. Infiltrate composed predominantly of lymphocytes.
2. Intraepidermal edema characteristic of hand, foot, and mouth disease.

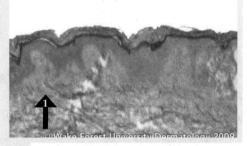

1. Superficial perivascular lymphohistiocytic infiltrate

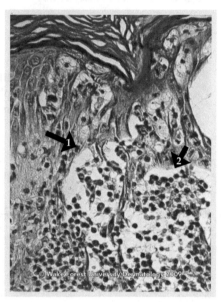

HISTOLOGICAL DIFFERENTIAL

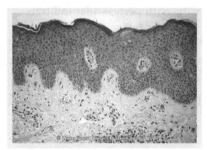

ACUTE SPONGIOTIC DERMATITIS

• More spongiosis in the epidermis
• Eosinophils present

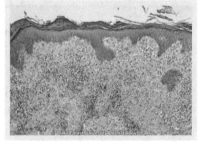

ERYTHEMA ANNULARE CENTRIFUGUM (EAC)

• Histopathology is similar, though EAC may have a denser, sleeve-like superficial perivascular infiltrate.

GOOD THINGS TO KNOW

• Diagnosis of a specific viral exanthem by histology is not always possible since findings are nonspecific; clinical correlation is necessary.
• Diffuse erythematous rashes in children: think viral etiology.
• Diffuse erythematous rashes in adults: think drug eruption.

Urticaria

Urticaria is not a disease, but transient, pruritic, edematous papules and plaques that are individually present for less than 24 hours. Outbreaks lasting less than 6 weeks are characterized as acute urticaria whereas outbreaks lasting longer than 6 weeks are characterized as chronic urticaria.

Histological Features

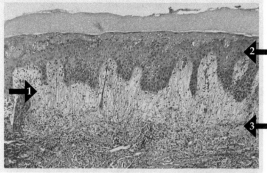

1. Edema in dermal papilla
2. Epidermis relatively unaffected
3. Superficial mixed perivascular infiltrate, primarily composed of lymphocytes and few eosinophils

1. Perivascular neutrophils
2. Perivascular erythrocytes
3. Dermal edema

Other Features:
• Mast cells and granulocytes within the interstitium
• Dilatation of venules

Histological Differential

ERYTHEMA MULTIFORME

• Perivascular inflammatory cell infiltrate predominantly composed of mononuclear cells
• Bulla formation with subepidermal separation
• Epidermal changes ranging from apoptotic keratinocytes to areas of epidermal necrosis

FIXED DRUG ERUPTION

• Dyskeratotic keratinocytes
• Interface vacuolar change and dermal edema
• Superficial perivascular lymphocytic infiltrate

Good Things To Know

If wheals do not disappear in under 24 hours, suspect urticarial vasculitis. Mast cells that have degranulated tend to look similar to lymphocytes.

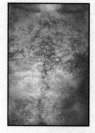

Epidemiology

• Approximately 20% of the population may be affected at some point in life.
• Etiologies include

- Drugs (commonly antipyretics and antibiotics
- Infections
- Foods
- External antigens
- Physical modalities (pressure, cold)
- Inflammatory disorders
• In most cases of urticaria, no identifiable etiology is found.

Pathophysiology

• The triple response is responsible for producing an urticarial lesion by
- Vasodilatation (erythema).
- Increased vascular permeability (wheal).
- Axon reflex (flare) occurs through stimulation of cutaneous nerve endings and release of substance P, a vasodilator, and causes the release of histamine from mast cells.

Clinical Features

• Urticarial lesions are hives that are recognized clinically as transient, pruritic, erythematous, edematous plaques that may display a central clearing.

Special Studies

• Biopsy when urticarial wheals have been present for >24 hours.
• CU Index (Chronic Urticaria Index) is available from a few reference laboratories.

Clinical Variants

• Immunologic urticaria
• Physical urticaria
• Non-immunologic urticaria
• Idiopathic (most common)

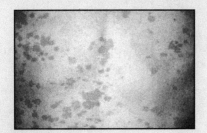

EPIDEMIOLOGY

- Common in young adults
- Can occur in 2% of population in temperate climates and 20% in tropical climates
- Predisposing factors:
    - Hyperhidrosis
    - Oily skin
    - Immunocompromise

PATHOPHYSIOLOGY

- In the presence of the above mentioned predisposing factors, *M. furfur* converts to the mycelial form that is responsible for clinical symptoms.
- Fatty acids in the skin are oxidized into dicarboxylic acids.
- Hypomelanosis results from inhibition of tyrosinase in epidermal melanocytes by dicarboxylic acid.

CLINICAL FEATURES

- Usually asymptomatic, but may have pruritus
- Well-demarcated round or oval-shaped dyspigmented macules that frequently coalesce
- Fine scale

SPECIAL STUDIES

- PAS stain can better visualize spores and hyphae.

CLINICAL VARIANTS

- None

TINEA VERSICOLOR

Tinea versicolor, also known as pityriasis versicolor, is a superficial fungal infection most commonly associated with overgrowth of *Malassezia furfur*.

HISTOLOGICAL FEATURES

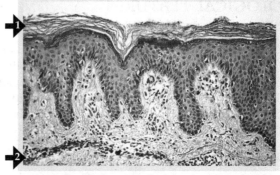

1. Hyperkeratosis
2. Minimal superficial perivascular lymphohistiocytic infiltrate

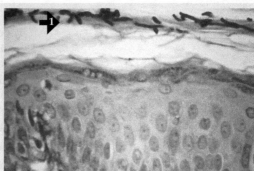

1. Fungal elements in stratum corneum ("spaghetti and meatballs")

HISTOLOGICAL DIFFERENTIAL

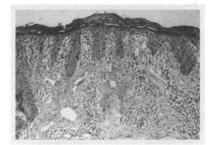

SEBORRHEIC DERMATITIS

- Caused by *M. furfur* and has a superficial perivascular pattern.
- Spongiosis is present.
- Mounds of parakeratosis in a perifollicular pattern.

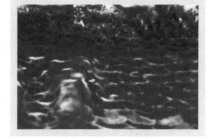

PITTED KERATOLYSIS

- Infectious elements seen within pits in stratum corneum.
- *Corynebacterium minutissimum* is causative agent and has a filamentous pattern, not a "spaghetti and meatballs" appearance.

GOOD THINGS TO KNOW

- Diagnosis can be confirmed by a KOH prep of scale.
- Woods lamp exam reveals yellow-green fluorescence of the lesions.

Pitted Keratolysis

Pitted keratolysis is a superficial infection most commonly caused by *Kytococcus sedentarius*. Common risk factors include prolonged occlusion of the feet and excessive heat and moisture. The diagnosis is often made clinically.

Histological Features

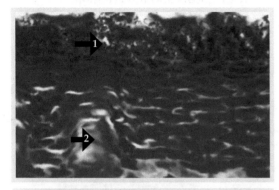

1. Infectious elements in pits in the stratum corneum
2. Sparse superficial perivascular inflammatory reaction

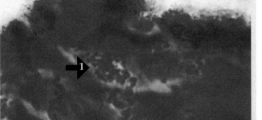

1. Infectious elements seen with H & E staining

Histological Differential

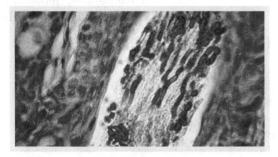

Tinea Pedis

• Fungal organisms in the stratum corneum stain positive for PAS.
• Tinea organisms are wider than filamentous bacteria in pitted keratolysis.

Good Things To Know

• Most labs do not routinely identify the causative agents of pitted keratolysis, so the pathology report may return as "diptheroids" or "normal skin flora."

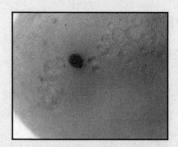

Epidemiology

• Occurs in children and adults of both genders.
• Most often occurs in adult males with sweaty feet making up 96% of all cases.
• Cases are more severe in tropical climates.

Pathophysiology

• The organism invades the stratum corneum, which is often softened by sweat and moisture.
• It also releases proteases that digest keratin and degrade the stratum corneum.

Clinical Features

• Numerous asymptomatic pits 1–2 mm or larger in size.
• Often occurs on pressure points such as the ventral aspect of the toe and the ball and heel of the foot.
• May also occur in the web spaces between the toes.
• Feet may have strong odor – 89% of cases.
• Patients may report socks stick to their feet – 70% of cases

Special Studies

• None

Clinical Variants

• None

EPIDEMIOLOGY

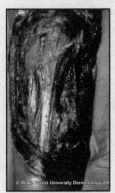

- Risk factors
  - Diabetes mellitus/diabetic ketoacidosis (most common)
  - Immuno-compromised host
    - Malignancy
    - Malnutrition
    - Trauma

PATHOPHYSIOLOGY

- Cutaneous involvement has two different pathways.
  - Mucorales are inhaled and can settle in the upper airways, lower airways, or gastrointestinal tract then disseminate to the skin.
  - Direct inoculation of spores into the skin, usually as a result of trauma.
- In all cases, infection can lead to blood vessel invasion, infarction, tissue necrosis and gangrene.

CLINICAL FEATURES

- Infected area initially erythematous and indurated and can progress to necrosis and black eschar formation.
- Eschars can become infected and develop cellulitis and abscesses.

SPECIAL STUDIES

- GMS
  - Stains fungi black against a green background
- PAS
  - Stains hyphae red

CLINICAL VARIANTS

- Rhinocerebral (most common)
- Cutaneous
- Pulmonary
- Gastrointestinal
- Isolated central nervous system
- Disseminated

MUCORMYCOSIS

Mucormycosis refers to a serious, uncommon fungal infection caused by Mucorales, which includes the genera *Absidia, Apophysomyceae, Mucor, Rhizomucor,* and *Rhizopus.* The poor prognosis (30–50% mortality rate for localized and higher rates in disseminated disease) of this infection necessitates early diagnosis and intervention.

HISTOLOGICAL FEATURES

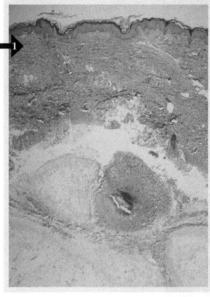

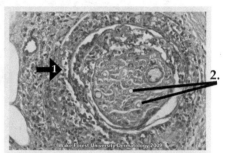

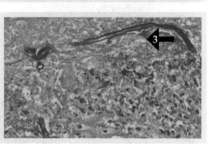

1. Sparse superficial perivascular infiltrate

1. Perivascular infiltrate
2. Multiple hyphae cut on end, occluding a blood vessel
3. Nonseptate, ribbon-like hyphae with branches at 90° angles

HISTOLOGICAL DIFFERENTIAL

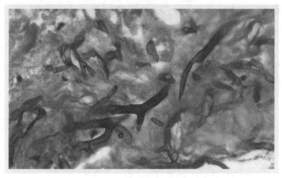

ASPERGILLOSIS

- Numerous septate hyphae branching at a 45° angle
- Differentiate by culture and histopathologic analysis of organism structure

GOOD THINGS TO KNOW

- Mucorales are often culture contaminants.

SUPERFICIAL PERIVASCULAR DERMATITIS
• INTERFACE DERMATITIS

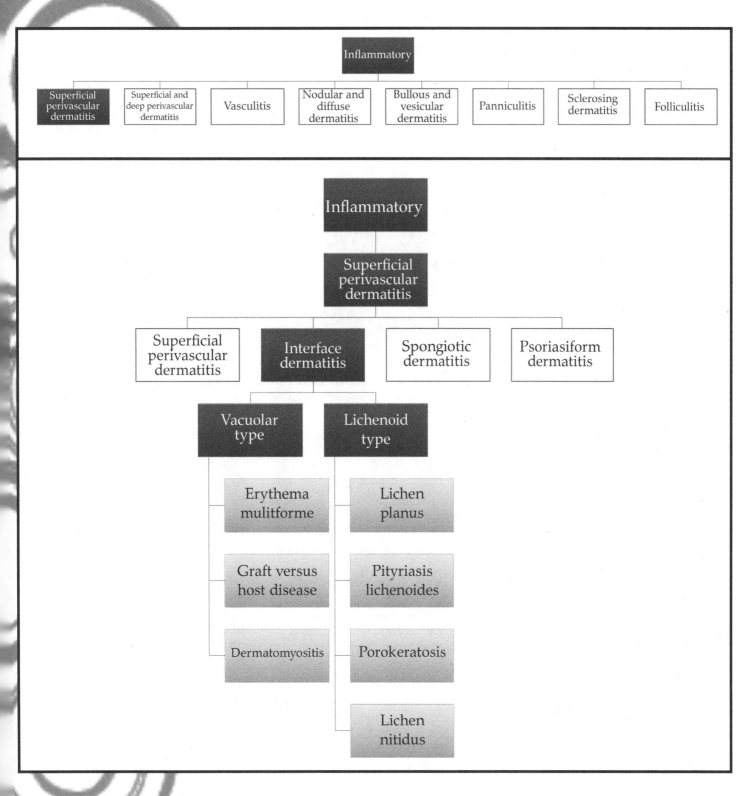

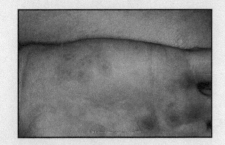

EPIDEMIOLOGY

- 50% occur in persons under 20 years
- More frequently seen in males than females

PATHOPHYSIOLOGY

- Believed to be an immune reaction directed at the skin following certain infections.
- EM following HSV infection is likely due to inflammation secondary to an autoimmune response from T cell recruitment to apoptotic cells containing HSV antigen.
- EM following other infections is less understood and likely have variable mechanisms.

CLINICAL FEATURES

- Sudden onset of symmetric erythematous skin lesions.
- Target lesions are the classical manifestation of erythema multiforme, and they are made up of three layers:

  – Zone 1= Dark and/ or blistered center ("bull's-eye" center)
  – Zone 2 = Surrounding pale zone
  – Zone 3= Outer ring of erythema

SPECIAL STUDIES

- PCR can be used to detect HSV.
- Frozen sections can be used to identify epidermal necrosis in severe TEN variant of EM.

CLINICAL VARIANTS

- EM Minor
- EM Major
- SJS/TEN

ERYTHEMA MULTIFORME

Erythema multiforme (EM) is an acute inflammatory skin disease that can develop from a number of causes, most commonly herpes simplex virus (HSV) infection, mycoplasma infection, or a drug reaction.

HISTOLOGICAL FEATURES

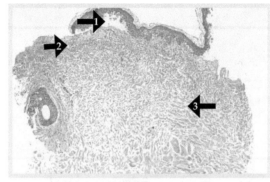

1. Subepidermal blister
2. Superficial perivascular mononuclear infiltrate
3. Dermal edema

1. Interface change with lymphocytes scattered along a vacuolated dermal–epidermal junction
2. Lymphocytic infiltrate
3. Dyskeratotic keratinocytes with focal epidermal necrosis

HISTOLOGICAL DIFFERENTIAL

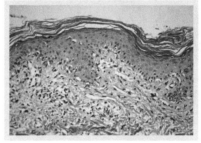

ACUTE GRAFT-VERSUS-HOST DISEASE

- Necrotic keratinocytes found in both
- More likely to have follicular involvement and sparse infiltrate
- Correlate clinically

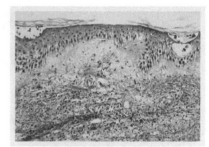

FIXED DRUG ERUPTION

- Necrotic keratinocytes found in both.
- More likely to have eosinophils.
- Interface vacuolar changes and dermal edema.
- Superficial and deep inflammation.

GOOD THINGS TO KNOW

- Since recurrent EM is caused by herpes simplex virus, frequent recurrences can be prevented by long-term use of anti-HSV medications.

Graft-Versus-Host Disease

Graft-versus-host disease (GVHD) results from donor immunocompetent T cells being introduced into a recipient that cannot reject them. The most common target tissues are liver, gastrointestinal, and skin.

Histological Features

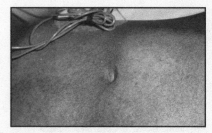

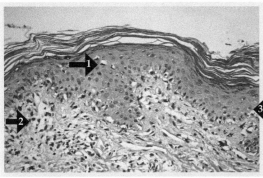

1. **Dyskeratotic keratinocyte**
2. **Superficial perivascular infiltrate**
3. **Interface dermatitis with vacuolar change**

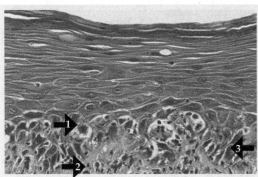

1. **Necrotic keratinocyte with adjacent lymphocytes (satellite cell necrosis)**
2. **Superficial infiltrate**
3. **Basal vacuolar changes**
Other features:
- **Graded severity based on histological findings:**
  - **Grade 1: Focal or diffuse vacuolar changes**
  - **Grade 2: Necrotic keratinocytes**
  - **Grade 3: Focal dermal–epidermal junction separation with vesicle formation**
  - **Grade 4: Bullae formation**

Histological Differential

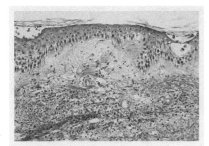

FIXED DRUG ERUPTION

- Necrotic keratinocytes
- Interface vacuolar changes
- Dermal edema
- Superficial and deep perivascular lymphocytes with eosinophils

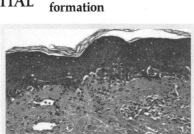

ERYTHEMA MULTIFORME

- Necrotic keratinocytes
- No satellite cell necrosiss
- Less likely to have follicular involvement
- Correlate clinically

Good Things To Know

- Staging (1-4) is based on degrees of clinical involvement.
- Grading (1-4) is based on histological features of skin biopsy.

Epidemiology
- Most often associated with allogenic bone marrow transplantations (BMT)
- Risk factors include
  - Unrelated, but matched donor
  - Related donor with one or more HLA mismatches
  - Older age of the donor or recipient

Pathophysiology
- GVHD develops from immunocompetent T cells recognizing foreign MHC complexes in the host.
- The major effectors in skin lesions are CD8+ T cells that utilize perforin and FasL to produce a cytotoxic effect.

Clinical Features
- Acute GVHD: Folliculocentric, morbilliform rash of abrupt onset that favors the distal extremities, pinnae, side of the neck, and upper back
- Chronic GVHD: Occurs more than 100 days post-transplant
  - Lichenoid: Erythematous or violaceous papules and plaques on the dorsal aspects of the hands, feet, forearms, and trunk
  - Sclerodermoid: Plaques of sclerosis that resemble morphea

Special Studies
- May use immunocytochemistry for HLA-DR, as expression on keratinocytes precedes changes morphologically

Clinical Variants
- Follicular
- Bullous
- Lichenoid
- Sclerodermoid

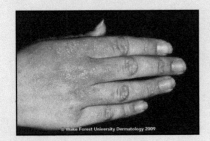

EPIDEMIOLOGY

- Unknown etiology.
- 2 peaks: one in childhood and one between 45–65.
- Female to male ratio is 6:1 in adult DM.

PATHOPHYSIOLOGY

- Thought to be immune-mediated from external factors (infection, malignancy, drugs) in genetically susceptible individuals

CLINICAL FEATURES

- Poikiloderma
  - Heliotrope rash
  - Gottran's papules
  - Gottran's sign
- Shawl sign or "V" sign–erythema over the chest and shoulders from photosensitivity
- Periungual telangectasia
- Calcinosis of subcutaneous/fascial tissues
- Proximal muscle weakness

SPECIAL STUDIES

- PAS-positive fibrinoid deposits
- DIF-positive along dermal–epidermal junction and along blood vessels

CLINICAL VARIANTS

- Amyopathic DM (DM sine myositis)
  - DM with cutaneous findings only
- Polymyositis
  - DM with muscular findings only

DERMATOMYOSITIS

Dermatomyositis (DM) is a systemic inflammatory disease that falls under idiopathic inflammatory myopathies. Diagnosis is made based on 5 criteria: cutaneous disease, muscle disease, symmetrical weakness, elevated levels of muscle enzymes, and abnormal electromyography.

HISTOLOGICAL FEATURES

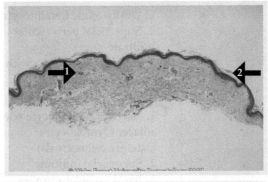

1. Sparse superficial perivascular infiltrate
2. Epidermal atrophy

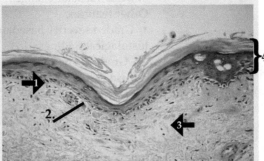

1. Interface change with vacuolar alteration of basal keratinocytes
2. Basement membrane degeneration
3. Dermal edema
4. Epidermal atrophy
Other features:
- Dermal mucin

HISTOLOGICAL DIFFERENTIAL

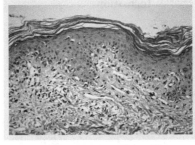

ACUTE GRAFT-VERSUS-HOST DISEASE

- Apoptotic keratinocytes
- Less infiltrate
- No dermal mucin

LUPUS ERYTHEMATOSUS (LE)

- DM can be identical to LE, but LE usually has more inflammation and vascular injury.
- Prominent interface change in epidermis and adnexal structures.
- No papillary dermal edema.

GOOD THINGS TO KNOW

- Vascular changes and immunofluorescence profile are valuable in differentiating DM from SLE.
- Adult DM is associated with internal malignancy in 30% of the cases.

LICHEN PLANUS

Lichen planus (LP) is the prototype of the lichenoid dermatoses and is characterized clinically by polygonal, flat-topped, violaceous papules and plaques. A band-like lymphocytic infiltrate is seen on histology with a "saw-tooth" pattern of the rete ridges.

HISTOLOGICAL FEATURES

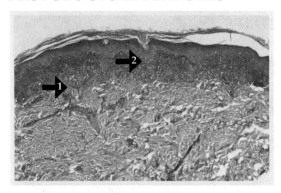

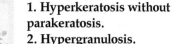

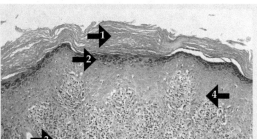

1. Lichenoid infiltrate of the upper dermis that may involve lower epidermis
2. Saw tooth rete ridges

1. Hyperkeratosis without parakeratosis.
2. Hypergranulosis.
3. Lichenoid infiltrate.
4. Irregular acanthosis causes the rete ridges to appear "saw-toothed."
Other features:
- Necrotic keratinocytes.
- Degeneration of the basal cell layer with vacuolization.

HISTOLOGICAL DIFFERENTIAL

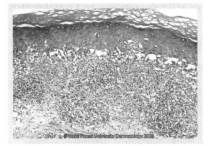

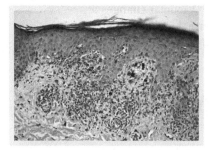

| LICHENOID DRUG REACTION | LICHEN PLANUS-LIKEKERATOSIS |

- Mucous membranes are typically spared.
- More likely to have eosinophils and plasma cells in the infiltrate with parakeratosis.

- May be identical to LP.
- Often is a solitary lesion with more parakeratosis, correlate clinically.

GOOD THINGS TO KNOW

- Associated drugs: ACE-inhibitors, thiazides, antimalarials, quinidine, and gold.
- Perform a punch biopsy to evaluate the entire dermis to rule out a deep inflammatory processes.

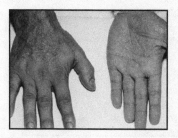

EPIDEMIOLOGY

- Incidence up to 1% of the adult population although wide variation among geographic location.
- Typical age of onset is 30–60 years.
- Oral involvement occurs in up to 75% of patients with skin manifestations.
- Associations with viral infection, medication, vaccine, and autoimmune disease.

PATHOPHYSIOLOGY

- Unknown etiology.
- Current studies suggest it is caused by a T-cell mediated autoimmune response to keratinocytes that were altered by various exposures, such as viral infection or drug use.

CLINICAL FEATURES

- Pruritic, purplish, polygonal, planar, papules or plaques ("the five Ps"). The lesions are covered with a very fine, white, reticulated scale known as "Wickham's striae."
- Often grouped on flexor surfaces (especially wrists), genitalia, and oral mucosa.

SPECIAL STUDIES

- None

CLINICAL VARIANTS

- Oral LP, nail LP, actinic LP, annular LP, bullous LP, hypertrophic LP, inverse LP, linear LP, lichen planopilaris, lichen planus pigmentosus, ulcerative LP, vulvovaginal LP

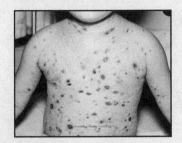

EPIDEMIOLOGY

• Usually presents in the first to third decades of life
• More common in males

PATHOPHYSIOLOGY

• Unknown etiology.
• Associated with various infectious agents (parvovirus B19), lymphomatoid papulosis, and immune-complex hypersensitivity.
• In situ polymerase chain reaction studies suggest it may be a form of T-cell lymphoproliferative disorder.

CLINICAL FEATURES

• In the acute form, lesions present as small edematous papules, pustules or vesicles with central necrosis and hemorrhagic crusting (PLEVA).
• In the chronic and milder form, lesions present as small red-brown papules with an overlying scale that generally involute and leave behind a hyperpigmented macule.
• Appears as crops located more commonly on the trunk and extremities.
• Usually asymptomatic, may be pruritic.

SPECIAL STUDIES

• Immunohistochemical analysis: PLEVA express CD2, CD3, and CD8 T cell antigens.

CLINICAL VARIANTS

• PLEVA
• PLC

PITYRIASIS LICHENOIDES

Pityriasis lichenoides (PL) is a self-limited dermatosis of unknown etiology. Cutaneous lesions present with various morphology ranging from the acute form, pityriasis lichenoides et varioliformis acuta (PLEVA) to the chronic form termed pityriasis lichenoides chronica (PLC).

HISTOLOGICAL FEATURES

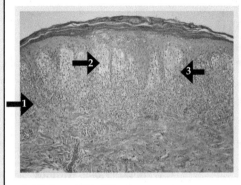

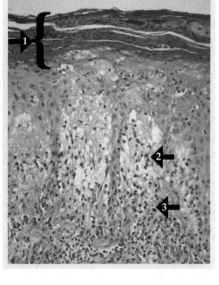

1. Lichenoid infiltrate
2. Vacuolar change at DEJ
3. Extravasation of RBCs

1. Parakeratosis
2. Erythrocytes
3. Dense lymphocytic infiltrate
Other features:
• PLEVA
  o Parakeratosis, spongiosis, intraepidermal lymphocytes, dyskeratosis, epidermal necrosis
  o Vacuolar changes at dermal–epidermal junction

o Dense perivascular lymphocytic infiltrate (lichenoid infiltrate) in papillary dermis that extends into the reticular dermis in a wedge-shaped pattern
  o Extravasation of erythrocytes
• PLC
  o Mild spongiosis and parakeratosis

HISTOLOGICAL DIFFERENTIAL

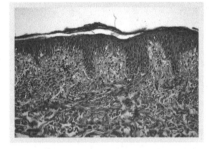

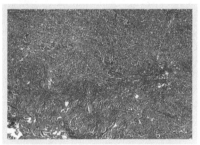

PITYRIASIS ROSEA
• Focal spongiosis and mounds of parakeratosis
• Lesser degree of epithelial injury
• Superficial sparse perivascular lymphohistiocytic infiltrate

LYMPHOMATOID PAPULOSIS
• Wedge-shaped dermal lymphocytic infiltrate
• Composed of pleomorphic or anaplastic lymphoid cells
• Atypical mitoses and CD30+ positive cells

GOOD THINGS TO KNOW
• PLEVA and PLC may appear simultaneously as they represent different spectrums of the disease.

Porokeratosis (PK)

Porokeratosis (PK) is a skin disease characterized by a thickening of the stratum corneum together with progressive centrifugal atrophy. The classic form of PK is porokeratosis of Mibelli which is a type usually appearing in childhood, but lesions may be present at birth, puberty or later.

Histological Features

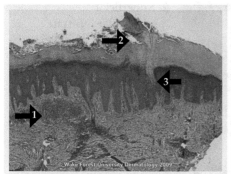

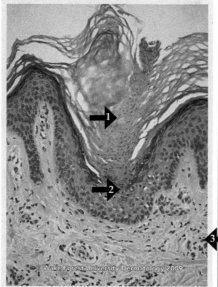

1. **Band-like lichenoid infiltrate**
2. **Column of parakeratosis**
3. **Hypogranulosis beneath cornoid lamella**

1. Cornoid lamella
2. Hypogranulosis and dyskeratosis underlying cornoid lamella
3. Superficial perivascular lymphocytic infiltrate

Histological Differential

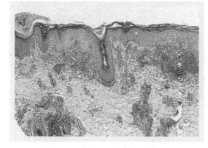

Lupus Erythematosus

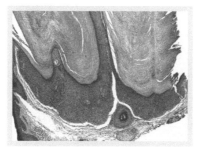

Actinic Keratosis

- Prominent interface change in epidermis and adnexal structures
- No cornoid lamella
- Perivascular lymphocytic infiltrate

- Areas of parakeratosis alternating with orthokeratosis
- No cornoid lamella

Good Things To Know

- When taking a biopsy of a suspected PK lesion, ensure that you biopsy a portion of the rim of the lesion to visualize cornoid lamellae.

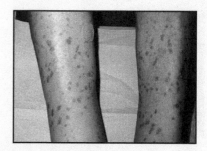

Epidemiology

- Disseminated superficial actinic porokeratosis (DSAP) is relatively common in the United States, whereas other forms are rare.

Pathophysiology

- May arise secondary to genetic predisposition, sporadically, or through induction by certain medications
- Association of porokeratosis with immunosuppression has also been described.

Clinical Features

- Lesions appear as sharply demarcated, annular, or serpiginous lesions with a hyperkeratotic ridge and an atrophic center.
- May appear as single or multiple lesions.

Special Studies

- PAS stains glycogen inclusions within cornoid lamella.

Clinical Variants

- Porokeratosis of Mibelli
- DSAP
- Porokeratosis punctata palmaris et plantaris
- Linear PK

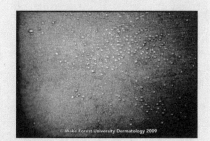

EPIDEMIOLOGY

• 4:1 male to female ratio.
• Greater incidence among African-Americans relative to Caucasians.
• Children and young adults are primarily affected.
• May be related to lichen planus and associated with psoriasis, juvenile idiopathic arthritis, Crohn's disease, amenorrhea.

PATHOPHYSIOLOGY

• Unknown

CLINICAL FEATURES

• Tiny flesh-colored papules appear on upper limbs, chest, abdomen, and genitals.
• Back, gums, and nails are also possible locations.

SPECIAL STUDIES

• Immunostains generally are not needed, but would show:
  - A large amount of CD4+ cells in contrast to CD8+ cells are seen.
  - High number of CD1+ cells.
  - KP1+ macrophages are seen and less lymphocytes show HECA-452.

CLINICAL VARIANTS

• None

LICHEN NITIDUS

Lichen nitidus is a rare inflammatory disease of the skin characterized by the chronic occurrence of localized uniform, pale-colored, flat-topped micropapules (pinpoint elevated lesions). It is asymptomatic, benign, and of unknown origin.

HISTOLOGICAL FEATURES

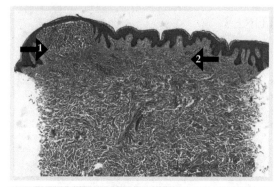

1. "Ball-in-claw" appearance
2. Superficial perivascular infiltrate

1. Interface dermatitis
2. Flattened epidermis
3. Lymphohistiocytic lichenoid infiltrate

Other Features:
• "Ball-in-claw" appearance
  - The ball is the infiltrate (made up of lymphocytes and histiocytes).
  - This is embedded in the claw (epidermal collarette).

HISTOLOGICAL DIFFERENTIAL

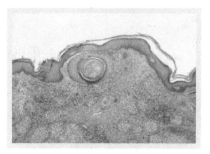

SARCOIDOSIS

• Granulomatous dermatitis
• No ball-in-claw appearance

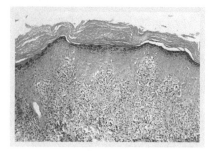

LICHEN PLANUS

• "Saw-toothed" rete ridges
• Band-like infiltrate in upper dermis
• Stains HECA-452+

GOOD THINGS TO KNOW

• In lichen nitidus, there are fewer lymphocytes that stain HECA-452+, whereas in lichen planus almost all cells are HECA-452+.

SUPERFICIAL PERIVASCULAR DERMATITIS

• SPONGIOTIC DERMATITIS

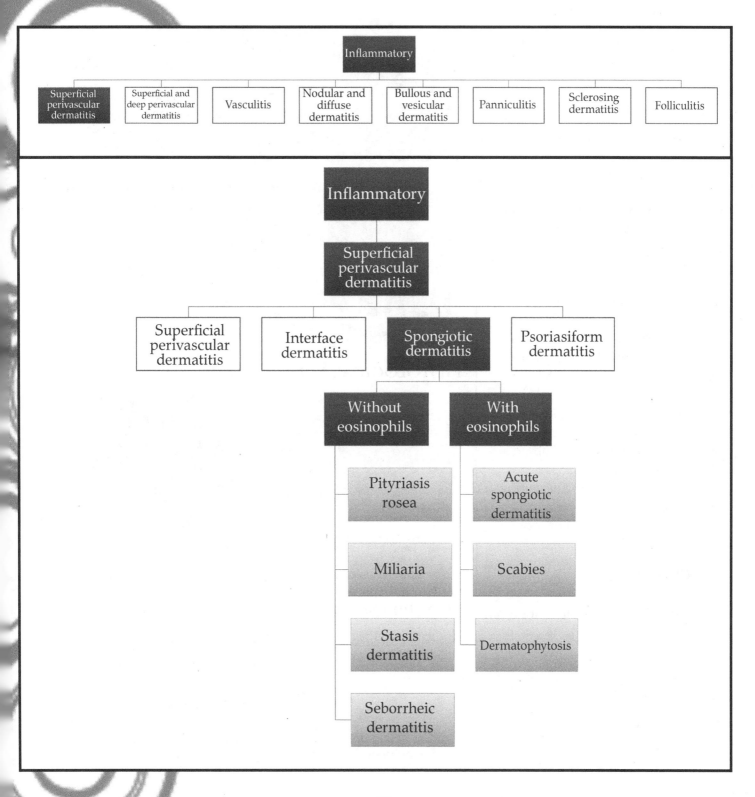

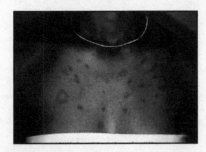

PITYRIASIS ROSEA

Pityriasis rosea (PR) is a self-limiting papulosquamous skin disease that begins with a characteristic scaly salmon-colored patch and spreads as scaling papules throughout the trunk and proximal limbs.

EPIDEMIOLOGY

• Although PR affects people of all ages, sexes, and ethnicities, 75% of cases are seen between the ages of 15 and 35.

PATHOPHYSIOLOGY

• Etiology is uncertain.
• Pityriasis rosea may be associated with primary infection and reactivation of Herpes Simplex Virus 6 and 7, and has histopathologic findings characteristic of viral infection.

CLINICAL FEATURES

• PR classically begins with a 2–10 cm salmon-colored oval "herald patch" with a collarette of scale on the inside border.
• Typically 1–2 weeks later, smaller scaly papules appear along Langer lines on the trunk and proximal limbs in a "Christmas tree" pattern.
• Some patients have pruritus during rash outbreak, but there are no other associated symptoms with the rash.

SPECIAL STUDIES

• PAS stain if needed to rule out tinea corporis

CLINICAL VARIANTS

•   None

HISTOLOGICAL FEATURES

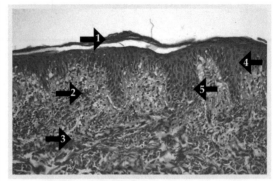

1. Mound of parakeratosis
2. Extravasated RBCs
3. Superficial perivascular lymphohistiocytic infiltrate
4. Slight spongiosis
5. Slight acanthosis

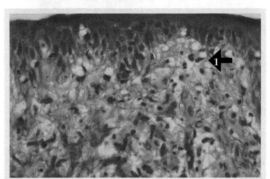

1. Extravasated erythrocytes in epidermis and dermal papilla

HISTOLOGICAL DIFFERENTIAL

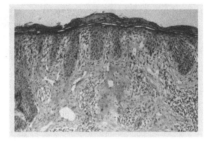

SEBORRHEIC DERMATITIS

• No extravasation of erythrocytes, mounds tend to be perifollicular.
• Clinical data may help as well.

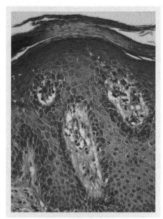

PSORIASIS

• Also has mounds of parakeratosis
• Neutrophils in the stratum corneum

GOOD THINGS TO KNOW

• The herald patch is often more spongiotic than other lesions.
• Spontaneously regresses after about 3–12 weeks.

Miliaria

Miliaria encompasses a family of common disorders of the eccrine sweat glands that is often associated with conditions of increased heat and humidity. It is also known as "heat rash" or "prickly heat." The four types of miliaria are differentiated by their clinical appearance and the location of the obstruction within the ducts.

Histological Features

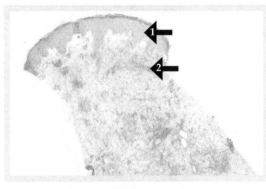

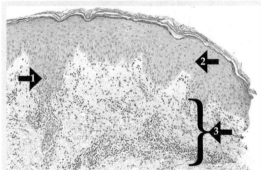

1. **Mild spongiosis**
2. **Superficial perivascular infiltrate**

~~~~~~~~~~~~~~~~~~~~~~~~~~~~~~

1. **Intraepidermal pustule**
2. **Mild spongiosis**
3. **Superficial perivascular infiltrate**

- Miliaria crystallina
  - Intracorneal or subcorneal vesicle arising from the acrosyringium of the sweat duct
- Miliaria rubra
  - Spongiotic intraepidermal vesicles
  - Chronic periductal inflammatory cell infiltrate in the papillary dermis and lower epidermis
- Miliaria pustulosa
  - Characteristics of miliaria rubra with a neutrophilic infiltrate
- Miliaria profunda
  - Substantial, periductal lymphocytic infiltrate
  - Spongiosis of the intra-epidermal duct

Histological Differential

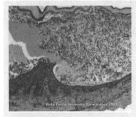

Subcorneal Pustular Dermatosis
- Intracorneal vesicle filled with neutrophils, but miliaria crystallina has a vesicle with more fluid and less neutrophils

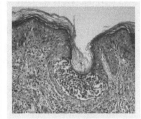

Erythema Toxicum
- Eosinophils are present.

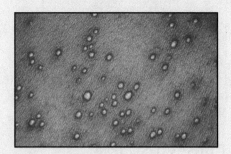

Epidemiology

- Miliaria crystallina and miliaria rubra are most common in infants.
- Commonly occurs in tropical or subtropical climates.
- Occurs in individuals of all races.

Pathophysiology

- Miliaria arises from obstruction of the sweat ducts.
- Leakage of sweat through the walls of the duct behind the block into the dermis or epidermis is responsible for production of miliaria.

Clinical Features

- Tiny 1–2 mm papules, vesicles, or pustules that may be confluent.
- Lesions may be itchy.
- Nonfollicular distribution.

Special Studies

- PAS stains positive for an amorphous, diastase-resistant material in the acrosyringium.

Clinical Variants

- Miliaria crystallina (sudamina)
- Miliaria rubra (prickly heat)
- Miliaria pustulosa
- Miliaria profunda (Mamillaria)

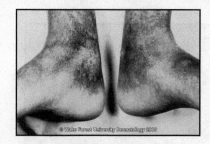

EPIDEMIOLOGY

• Predisposing factors: history of varicose veins, congestive heart failure, obesity, surgery, trauma and/or thrombosis
• Precipitating factors: standing for long periods of time, pregnancy, and other causes of venous hypertension

PATHOPHYSIOLOGY

• Incompetent deep vein valves lead to a backflow of blood causing pressure, oxygen content and flow rate to increase and produce changes in the surrounding dermis and epidermis.
• Hemosiderin deposits from degraded hemoglobin in extravasated red blood cells cause pigmentary changes.

CLINICAL FEATURES

• Changes include edema, hyperpigmentation, and fibrosis.
• Typically seen above the medial malleolus.
• Common complication: ulcer formation.

SPECIAL STUDIES

• Hemosiderin deposits can be stained with Prussian blue and Perl's potassium ferrocyanide.

CLINICAL VARIANTS

• Acroangiodermatitis (pseudo Kaposi sarcoma)

STASIS DERMATITIS

Stasis dermatitis is a classic eczematous dermatitis that commonly affects the lower extremities secondary to chronic venous insufficiency.

HISTOLOGICAL FEATURES

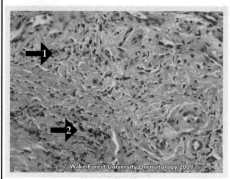
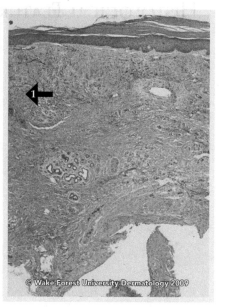

1. Extravasation of erythrocytes
2. Hemosiderin deposits and macrophages

1. Vascular proliferation
Other features:
• **Spongiosis**
• **Superficial perivascular infiltrate**

HISTOLOGICAL DIFFERENTIAL

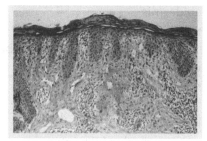
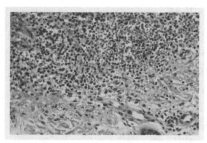

SEBORRHEIC DERMATITIS   PIGMENTED PURPURIC DERMATOSIS

• Spongiosis
• Usually more psoriasiform in appearance
• No extravasated erythrocytes
• No hemosiderin deposits
• No vascular proliferation

• Extravasated erythrocytes
• Hemosiderin-laden macrophages
• No vascular proliferation

GOOD THINGS TO KNOW

• Lobular arrangement of blood vessels, extravasated erythrocytes, and hemosiderin deposition are common findings.

Seborrheic Dermatitis

Seborrheic dermatitis (SD) is a common benign papulosquamous condition involving greasy, yellowish scales on the scalp and face of infants and middle-aged adults. Its exact cause is unknown, but may be associated with yeast over-growth and/or an altered immune response.

Histological Features

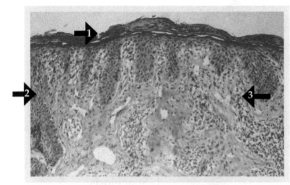

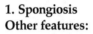

1. Neutrophils in a mound of parakeratosis
2. Acanthosis
3. Perivascular lymphocytic infiltrate

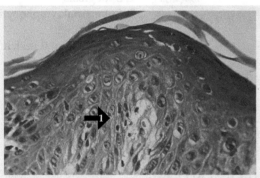

1. Spongiosis
Other features:
• Perifollicular parakeratotic mounds
• Yeast with KOH stain

Histological Differential

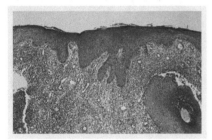

Tinea Capitis

• Absence of hyphae on KOH stain

Psoriasis

• Both have focal parakeratosis.
• Neutrophils in stratum corneum.
• Only SD has the spongiform pattern.

Good Things To Know

• Generalized, severe SD in infants may be a sign of Leiner's disease, a dangerous condition characterized by SD, diarrhea, failure to thrive, and frequent infections.

Epidemiology

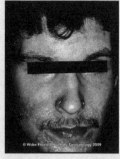

• Affects 3% of general population
• Bimodal peak: 10% of infants in first 3 months; adults, between 18–40 years old
• Also seen in immunocompromised patients
• More common in winter months and in patients with little sun exposure

Pathophysiology

• Highly associated with increases of the malassezia yeast *Pityrosporon ovale*.
• SD in HIV patients may be caused by an abnormal immune response to *P. ovale.*
• SD in infants may be caused by excess sebaceous secretions.

Clinical Features

• Greasy, yellow non-adherent scales on areas with high sebaceous secretions
• Moderate itching and erythema
• Location:
  – Infants - "cradle cap": scalp, eyebrows, nasolabial folds, flexural and diaper areas
  – Adults - hair-bearing regions: scalp, face, chest and back
  – Immunocompromised - diffuse involvement.

Special Studies

• Although SD is predominately a clinical diagnosis, a skin biopsy is the only way to confirm.

Clinical Variants

• None

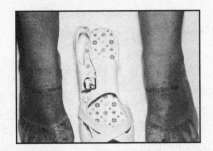

EPIDEMIOLOGY

• ASD is one of the most common dermatologic diagnoses
• 9% of visits to dermatologists are for dermatitis

PATHOPHYSIOLOGY

• Fluid from vasculature passes to the dermis and then the epidermis

CLINICAL FEATURES

• The primary acute symptom change is erythema with vesicles and crust
• Pruritus

SPECIAL STUDIES

• PAS stain to rule out Dermatophytosis if neutrophils are identified in the stratum corneum

CLINICAL VARIANTS

• Found in various entities, including
   - Atopic dermatitis
   - Contact dermatitis
   - Nummular dermatitis
   - Dyshidrotic eczema

ACUTE SPONGIOTIC DERMATITIS

Acute spongiotic dermatitis (ASD) is an inflammatory skin disorder due to exposure to various irritants and antigens.

HISTOLOGICAL FEATURES

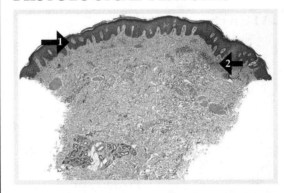

1. Intraepidermal vesicle
2. Superficial perivascular lymphocytic infiltrate

1. Spongiosis
2. Superficial lymphocytic infiltrate
3. Intraepidermal vesicle

Other features:
• Eosinophils are commonly present in the dermal infiltrate and epidermis.

HISTOLOGICAL DIFFERENTIAL

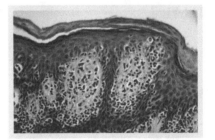

MYCOSIS FUNGOIDES

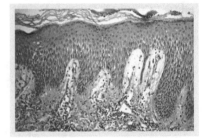

DERMATOPHYTOSES

• Exocytosis of mononuclear cells out of proportion to the amount of spongiosis
• Lymphocytes with atypical cerebriform nuclei

• Fungal hyphae and/or neutrophils in stratum corneum

GOOD THINGS TO KNOW

• A spongiotic dermatitis can be superimposed over other eruptions if patients apply topical treatments to which they are allergic.

SCABIES

Scabies is an infestation of the epidermis caused by the itch mite *Sarcoptes scabiei*. Lesions are intensely pruritic and present as linear burrows with a small vesicle at the blind end.

HISTOLOGICAL FEATURES

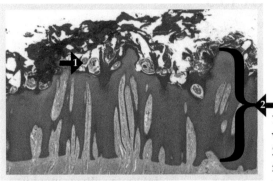

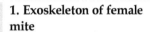

1. **Mite and products within the stratum corneum**
2. **Irregular acanthosis and focal spongiosis**

1. **Exoskeleton of female mite**

Other features:
- **Perivascular infiltrate of lymphocytes and eosinophils in the dermis**

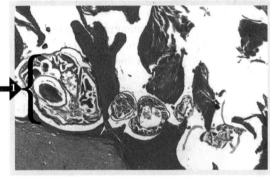

HISTOLOGICAL DIFFERENTIAL

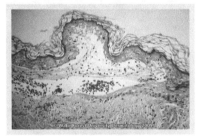

ARTHROPOD BITE

- No organisms in stratum corneum
- Superficial crust, spongiosis, and/or focal necrosis
- Wedge-shaped perivascular mixed infiltrate with eosinophils

CONTACT DERMATITIS

- Normal stratum corneum
- Spongiosis with intraepidermal vesicles
- Eosinophils in dermal infiltrate

GOOD THINGS TO KNOW

- If left untreated the infestation may last for many years, with the number of mites decreasing over time in an immunocompetent host.

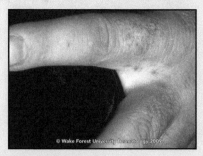

EPIDEMIOLOGY

- Affects all socioeconomic classes
- Seen in children, young adults, and elderly bedridden patients
- More prevalent in urban areas and overcrowded regions
- Transmission via skin to skin contact and fomites

PATHOPHYSIOLOGY

- Female mites tunnel and burrow into the epidermis, lay their eggs, and deposit feces in the stratum corneum.
- Sensitization to the foreign material causes an immediate and delayed hypersensitivity reaction.

CLINICAL FEATURES

- The pathognomonic lesion consists of burrows with a small vesicle at the blind end.
- Small erythematous excoriated papules.
- Predilection for web spaces of the fingers and toes, flexor surfaces of wrists, and lateral and palmar aspects of fingers.
- Intensely pruritic, typically worse at night.
- Areas of excoriation, lichenification, irritant dermatitis, or secondary infection are common.

SPECIAL STUDIES

- Dermoscopy: "jet-with-contrail" image
- Superficial epidermal shave biopsy will reveal the mite or its products

CLINICAL VARIANTS

- None

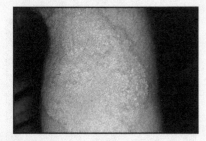

EPIDEMIOLOGY

• Infections are caused by parasitic fungi from the *Epidermophyton*, *Microsporum*, and *Trichophyton* genera.
• 30 to 70% of adult carriers are asymptomatic.
• *Trichophyton rubrum* is the most common cause of tinea pedis, onychomycosis, tinea cruris, and tinea corporis worldwide.

PATHOPHYSIOLOGY

• Dermatophytes grow in the presence of keratin (present in the stratum corneum, nail bed, and hair) which is degraded by keratinases.
• Temperature, humidity, and injury to infected areas influence the penetration of dermatophytes into the stratum corneum.
• Host-response to metabolic by-products of proteinase activity results in inflammation.

CLINICAL FEATURES

• Annular crusting and peripheral scaling can be seen at sites of infection
• Onychomycosis: thickening, discoloration, pain in the nail plate

SPECIAL STUDIES

• Periodic acid-Schiff (PAS) stain
• Grocott methenamine silver (GMS) stain
• Wood's lamp
• Fungal cultures – Sabouraud's glucose medium

CLINICAL VARIANTS

• None

DERMATOPHYTOSES

Dermatophytes are a group of fungi that affect the skin, hair, and nails. The most common infections include tinea pedis, tinea cruris, tinea facei, tinea capitis, and onychomycosis (tinea unguum)

HISTOLOGICAL FEATURES

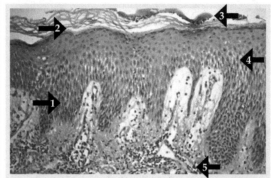

1. Epidermal hyperplasia
2. Orthokeratosis
3. Hyphae
4. Spongiosis
5. Superficial perivascular infiltrate with eosinophils

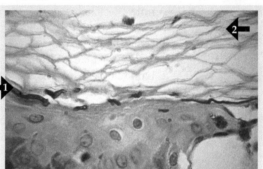

1. Fungal elements in stratum corneum
2. Orthokeratosis

Other features:
• Exocytosis of neutrophils in stratum corneum, can form spongiform pustule

HISTOLOGICAL DIFFERENTIAL

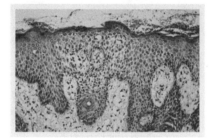

ALLERGIC CONTACT DERMATITIS

• No fungal elements in stratum corneum
• More spongiosis
• Also may have eosinophils

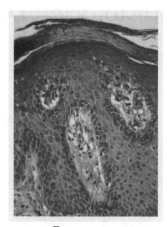

PSORIASIS
• No fungal elements in stratum corneum
• Parakeratosis
• Neutrophils in stratum corneum

GOOD THINGS TO KNOW

• Dermatophytoses can mimic various inflammatory conditions; therefore, testing for fungal infection in the presence of uncertain inflammatory dermatoses is wise.

SUPERFICIAL PERIVASCULAR DERMATITIS

• PSORIASIFORM DERMATITIS

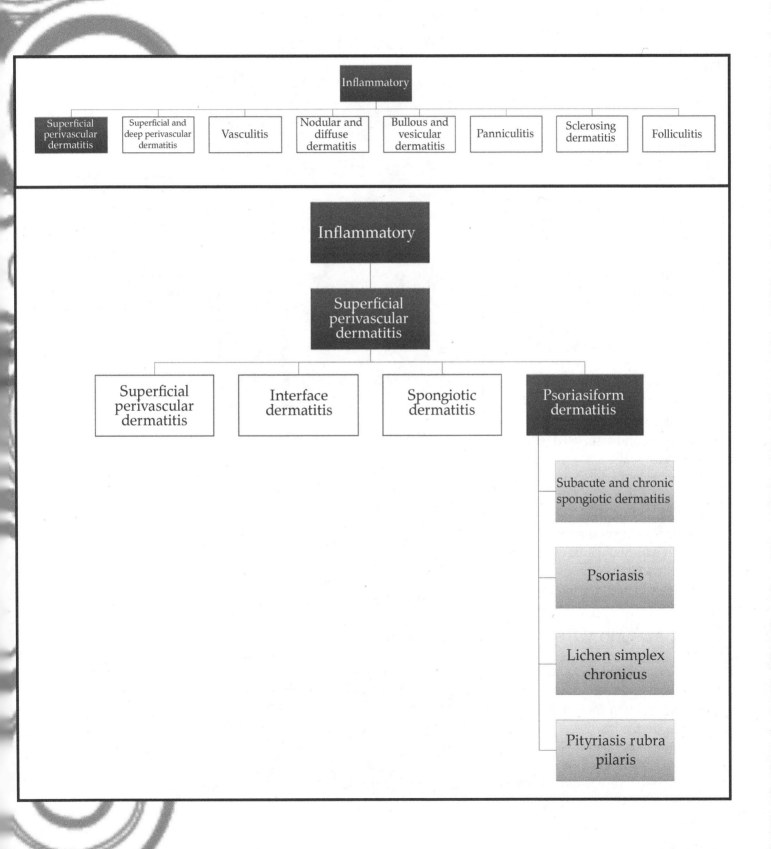

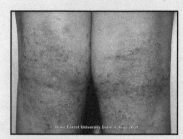

EPIDEMIOLOGY

• Spongiotic dermatoses are some of the most commonly treated skin disorders.

PATHOPHYSIOLOGY

• Orderly progression of changes:
  - Acute: an initial inflammatory reaction in which epidermal edema is a prominent feature.
  - Subacute: some edema may still be present, but much has moved to the stratum corneum in the form of scale crust.
  - Chronic: the edema has resolved, but the epidermis is markedly thickened due to hyperproliferation of keratinocytes and some dermal changes are present as well.

CLINICAL FEATURES

• Dependent on disease entity.
• Subacute: most lesions are erythematous and associated with crust or crust scale.
• Chronic: lichenification, pruritus.

SPECIAL STUDIES

• Routine staining of the scale associated with spongiotic dermatitis followed by a Gram stain can identify the presence of bacterial infection.

CLINICAL VARIANTS

• In various entities, including
  - Xerotic dermatitis.
  - Allergic/irritant contact dermatitis.
  - Atopic dermatitis.
  - Nummular dermatitis.
  - Lichen simplex chronicus and prurigo nodularis are chronic forms of spongiotic dermatitis.

SUBACUTE AND CHRONIC SPONGIOTIC DERMATITIS

Subacute and chronic spongiotic dermatitis represent a spectrum of histological changes seen in many inflammatory skin diseases. Some features may provide important clues to reach a specific diagnosis.

HISTOLOGICAL FEATURES

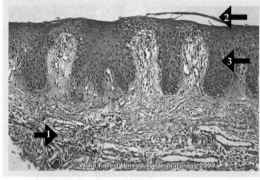

1. **Lymphohistiocytic dermal infiltrate**
2. **Parakeratosis**
3. **Spongiosis**

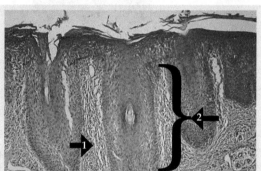

1. **Vertically streaked collagen in papillary dermis**
2. **Epidermal hyperplasia**

• Histological changes parallel the severity of the clinical disease
• Subacute:
  - Variable spongiosis and parakeratosis
  - Lymphohistiocytic infiltration of dermis
• Chronic:
  - Minimal spongiosis
  - Hyperkeratosis with focal parakeratosis
  - Hypergranulosis
  - Epidermal hyperplasia
  - Vertically streaked collagen in papillary dermis

HISTOLOGICAL DIFFERENTIAL

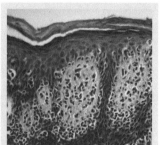

MYCOSIS FUNGOIDES

• Exocytosis of mononuclear cells out of proportion to the amount of spongiosis
• Lymphocytes with atypical cerebriform nuclei

GOOD THINGS TO KNOW

• The location of lesions may correlate with the type of spongiotic dermatitis.

Psoriasis

Psoriasis is a papulosquamous disorder composed of well-demarcated, erythematous papules and plaques with overlying silvery scale.

Histological Features

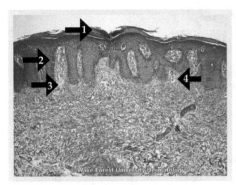
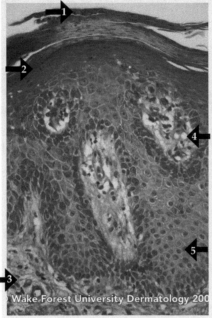

1. Hyperparakeratosis
2. Elongation of rete ridges
3. Superficial perivascular infiltrate
4. Dermal edema

1. Neutrophils in stratum corneum (Munro's microabscesses)
2. Decreased granular layer
3. Superficial perivascular infiltrate
4. Tortuous capillary
5. Acanthosis

Histological Differential

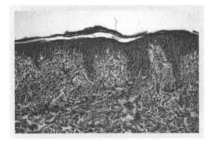

PITYRIASIS ROSEA

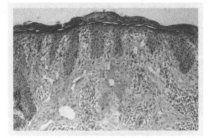

SEBORRHEIC DERMATITIS

• Parakeratosis in mounds is similar to psoriasis, but neutrophils are absent in pityriasis rosea.
• Granular layer is absent instead of decreased.
• Extravasated red blood cells.

• Parakeratosis is focal instead of confluent.
• Neutrophils collect at the tips of dilated follicular openings.

Good Things To Know

• Diagnosis is mainly clinical and biopsy is usually not required.
• Rule out fungal infection via PAS stain.

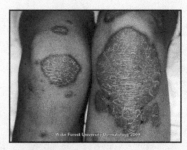

Epidemiology

• 1–2% of American population affected
• Streptococcal infection may precede eruption of guttate plaques.
• Plaques may occur in response to trauma (Koebner phenomenon), emotional stress or drugs.

Pathophysiology

• Psoriatic lesions develop due to interactions between inflammatory cells and keratinocytes, leading to increased epidermal proliferation rates that cause cells to transit from the basal cell layer to the top of the stratum corneum in a decreased amount of time.
• The exact mechanism of how this occurs is not currently known.
• There is a common notion of a genetic predisposition to psoriasis.

Clinical Features

• Preferential involvement of scalp, extensor surfaces of arms and legs, and sacral-gluteal region.
• Intertriginal involvement lacks the characteristic scale.
• Nail involvement (pitting, onycholysis, oil-spots).
• Arthritis may be present in up to 15% of psoriasis patients
• Auspitz's sign: punctate hemorrhages in areas where scale is removed.

Special Studies

• PAS with diastase to rule out fungal infection.

Clinical Variants

• Psoriasis vulgaris (most common)
• Pustular psoriasis
• Erythrodermic psoriasis
• Guttate psoriasis
• Inverse/flexural psoriasis

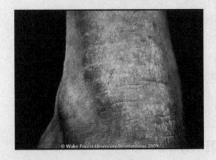

EPIDEMIOLOGY

- Reportedly more common in women.
- Generally seen in adults over 20 years of age.
- Some patients have an underlying emotional or psychiatric conditions.
- In some patients, it is caused by a nervous habit or sign of stress.

PATHOPHYSIOLOGY

- Itch–scratch–itch cycle
  - Skin is hypersensitive to any stimuli (touch, warmth, sweat).
  - Results in an abnormal scratching sensation of lichenified skin that is not provoked on normal skin.
- Itching and pruritus occur first, then the rash appears.

CLINICAL FEATURES

- Thickened plaques of lichenification
- Accentuated skin markings
- Progressive hyperpigmentation
- Common sites: posterior neck, flexural areas, lower extremities, genital area

SPECIAL STUDIES

- Patch test may rule out ACD.
- PAS stain can be done if tinea is suspected.

CLINICAL VARIANTS

- None

LICHEN SIMPLEX CHRONICUS

Lichen simplex chronicus is an inflammatory process associated with thickening of the skin due to repetitive mechanical trauma.

HISTOLOGICAL FEATURES

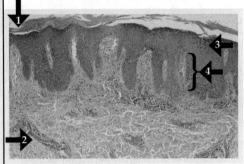

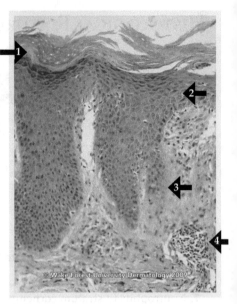

1. Hyperkeratosis
2. Perivascular lymphocytic infiltrate
3. Hypergranulosis
4. Elongation of rete ridges

1. Hyperkeratosis
2. Lack of spongiosis
3. Vertically oriented collagen in papillary dermis
4. Perivascular lymphocytic infiltrate

Other features:
- Excoriations appear as punctate ulcerations surrounded by a necrotic superficial dermis and neutrophilic infiltrate.

HISTOLOGICAL DIFFERENTIAL

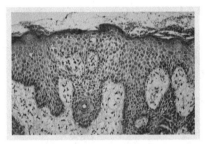

ALLERGIC CONTACT DERMATITIS (ACD)

- Prominent spongiosis
- Superficial dermal infiltrate composed of lymphocytes, macrophages, and Langerhans cells
- Eosinophils in dermis

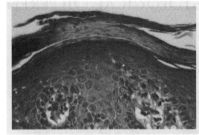

PSORIASIS

- Neutrophils in stratum corneum
- Parakeratosis, acanthosis with elongation of rete ridges
- Decreased granular layer
- Edematous dermal papillae
- Superficial perivascular mononuclear infiltrate

GOOD THINGS TO KNOW

- Lichenification can develop secondary to any pruritic or eczematous dermatitis.

Pityriasis Rubra Pilaris

Pityriasis rubra pilaris (PRP) is a papulosquamous disease of unknown etiology characterized by reddish orange scaly plaques, palmoplantar keratoderma, keratotic follicular papules, and islands of normal skin. It can mimic psoriasis both clinically and histologically.

Histological Features

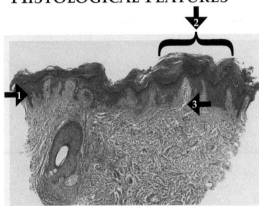

1. Psoriasiform dermatitis
2. Alternating orthokeratosis and parakeratosis in both the vertical and horizontal directions resulting in a "checkerboard" pattern
3. Superficial perivascular lymphocytic infiltrate

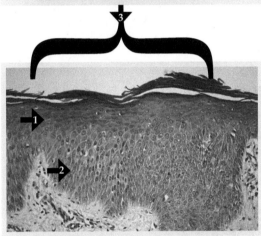

1. Hypergranulosis
2. Acanthosis
3. Alternating layers of orthokeratosis and para-keratosis: "checkerboard" pattern

Other features:
• Hair follicles are dilated and filled with a dense, horny plug.

Histological Differential

Psoriasis

• Neutrophils in the stratum corneum
• Tortuous capillaries in the dermal papillae
• Regular elongation of rete ridges

Good Things To Know

• One of the main keys to histological diagnosis is the checkerboard pattern in the stratum corneum.

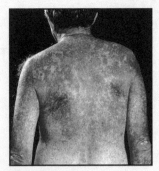

Epidemiology

• PRP has been reported all over the world, in all races, and affects men and women equally.
• Bimodal distribution: peaking in the first and fifth decades.

Pathophysiology

• Unknown
• May be associated with Vitamin A deficiency or physical trauma

Clinical Features

• Eruption of red to orange follicular hyperkeratotic papules which spread in a cephalocaudal pattern.
• Palms and soles become hyperkeratotic and develop an orange hue, which is often very painful and disabling when fissures develop.
• Nail involvement demonstrates yellow–brown discolorations with splinter hemorrhages and nail plate thickening.

Special Studies
• None

Clinical Variants

• Type I (Classic Adult)
  - Most common, >50% of all cases
• Type II (Atypical Adult)
• Type III (Classic Juvenile)
• Type IV (Circumscribed Juvenile)
• Type V (Atypical Juvenile)
• Type VI (HIV-associated)

Superficial & Deep Perivascular Dermatitis

- LYMPHOHISTIOCYTIC INFILTRATE
- MIXED-CELL INFILTRATE

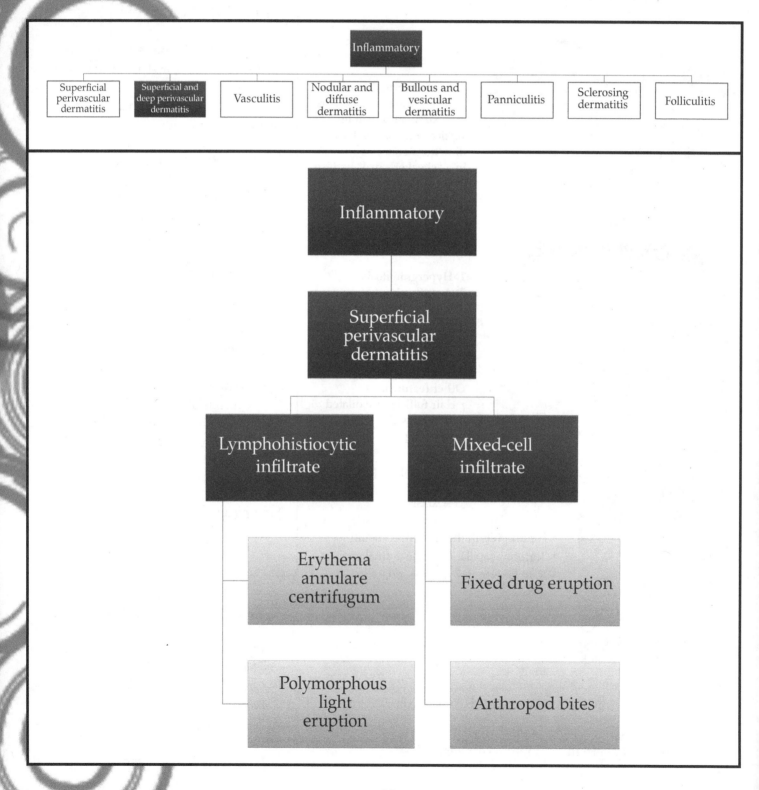

Erythema Annulare Centrifugum

Erythema annulare centrifugum (EAC), also known as superficial or deep gyrate erythema, is a figurate erythema that consists of migrating annular or arcuate erythematous plaques.

Histological Features

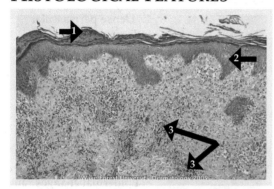

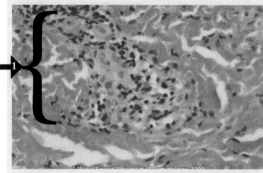

1. Parakeratosis.
2. Spongiosis.
3. Dense infiltrate of lymphocytes surround the superficial venous plexus in a "coat-sleeve" distribution.

1. Dense lymphocytic infiltrate.
• Focal spongiosis and parakeratosis in the expanding border.
• Edema of the papillary dermis.
• In the deep variant, the lymphocytic infiltrate is also present in the deep vascular plexuses, but superficial and deep involvement should raise the possibility of lupus erythematosus.

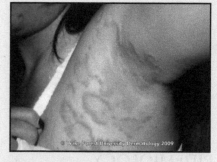

Epidemiology

• Estimated incidence is 1 in 100,000 per year.
• Most cases are idiopathic.
• Peak age of onset is in the 50s.

Pathophysiology

• Unknown pathomechanism
• It is thought to be a hypersensitivity reaction to an antigen or disease state.
  - Is associated with foods, certain drugs (penicillin, cimetidine), illness (malignancy, SLE, Sjogren's syndrome), and infection (bacterial, rickettsial, viral, and fungal).

Clinical Features

• Lesions begin as papules that expand centrifugally with central clearing.
• In the superficial variant a collarette of trailing scale is found on the inner margin on the expanding edge of erythema.
• Usually found on the trunk, thighs, or legs.
• Lesions may be pruritic.

Special Studies

• None

Histological Differential

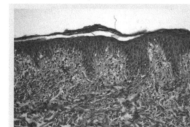

Secondary Syphilis
• Perivascular inflammatory infiltrate in a "coat-sleeve" distribution
• Presence of numerous plasma cells and histiocytes
• Vascular changes: swollen intimal and endothelial cells.

Pityriasis Rosea (PR)
• Perivascular inflammatory infiltrate
• Subacute spongiotic dermatitis with focal parakeratosis
• May have additional features of hyperkeratosis and acanthosis

Clinical Variants

• Nones

Good Things To Know

• While normally there is no epidermal change, there can be some parakeratosis and spongiosis, and rarely microvesiculation is also present.
• Histiocytes and eosinophils occasionally present in the inflammatory infiltrate.

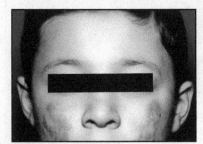

EPIDEMIOLOGY

• 2–3 times more common in females
• Affects all skin phototypes, but more common in fair-skinned individuals with skin types I–IV

PATHOPHYSIOLOGY

• Multifactorial etiology
• Eruption induced by UV radiation exposure (UVA and UVB)
• Delayed type hypersensitivity (DTH) response consisting of UV radiation-induced dermal cellular infiltration, cytokine production and adhesion molecule expression

CLINICAL FEATURES

• Sudden onset on sun-exposed skin (upper chest and arms)
• Lesions vary from erythematous and pruritic plaques, patches, or vesicles
• Typically subsides over 7–10 days without scarring

SPECIAL STUDIES

• Monochromatic or broad-spectrum irradiation skin tests to induce the classic eruption in settings of diagnostic uncertainty

CLINICAL VARIANTS

• African Americans: variant with pinpoint papules (1–2 mm) on sun-exposed areas, sparing the face and flexural surfaces
• Juvenile spring eruption: PMLE confined to the ears

POLYMORPHOUS LIGHT ERUPTION

Polymorphous light eruption (PMLE) is an idiopathic photodermatosis that is characterized by recurrent delayed reactions to sunlight. Reactions vary and range from erythematous papules, papulovesicles and plaques to erythema multiforme-like lesions on sun-exposed skin surfaces.

HISTOLOGICAL FEATURES

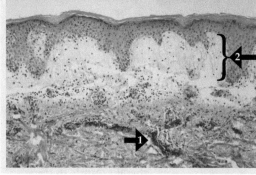

1. **Dense perivascular inflammatory infiltrate**
2. **Papillary dermal edema**

1. **Perivascular inflammatory infiltrate**
2. **Dermal blood vessel**

Other features:
• **Epidermal changes range from normal to spongiosis and acanthosis depending on the age of the lesion.**
• **Superficial and deep perivascular and periadnexal lymphohistiocytic inflammatory infiltrate.**
• **Occasional eosinophils and rare neutrophils may be found.**

HISTOLOGICAL DIFFERENTIAL

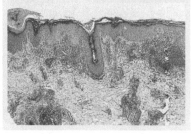

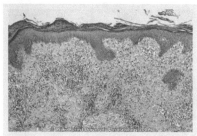

CUTANEOUS LUPUS ERYTHEMATOSUS
• Prominent interface change in the epidermis and adnexal structures.
• Apoptotic keratinocytes are often seen.
  - No papillary dermal edema
  - Dermal mucin deposition

SUPERFICIAL GYRATE ERYTHEMA (ERYTHEMA ANNULARE CENTRIFUGUM)

• Spongiosis and parakeratosis
• Dense perivascular lymphocytic infiltrate in superficial dermis
  - No neutrophilic component

GOOD THINGS TO KNOW

• PMLE is often discovered incidentally because many patients do not visit a physician.
• Actinic prurigo and hydroa vacciniforme are two other forms of photodermatosis.

ARTHROPOD BITES

Arthropod bites produce an acute localized inflammatory wheal that is often followed by a subacute or chronic inflammatory papule. The degree of inflammation correlates with the extent of the immune response to deposited foreign substances.

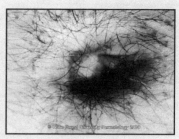

HISTOLOGICAL FEATURES

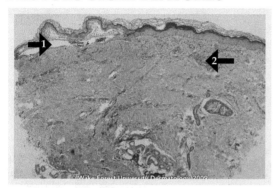

1. **Intraepidermal vesicle at bite site**
2. **Wedge-shaped mixed inflammatory infiltrate**

1. **Intraepidermal vesicle**
2. **Lymphocytes and eosinophils**

Other features:
- **Superficial crust, spongiosis, and/or focal necrosis.**
- **Edema of the papillary dermis.**
- **Vesiculobullous eosinophilic lesions may also occur.**

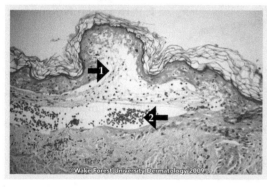

HISTOLOGICAL DIFFERENTIAL

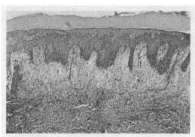

URTICARIA

- Papillary dermal edema
- Sparse lymphocytic perivascular infiltrate
- Dilated venules
- Eosinophils not prominent

LYMPHOMATOID PAPULOSIS

- Wedge-shaped superficial and deep dermal lymphocytic infiltrate
- Composed of pleomorphic or anaplastic lymphoid cells
- Atypical mitoses

GOOD THINGS TO KNOW

- An exaggerated bite response has been reported in immunocompromised patients, particularly in leukemia, lymphoma and HIV patients.

EPIDEMIOLOGY

- Most common in temperate climates during the summer
- Increased risk associated with poor personal hygiene and crowded or open-air living quarters
- Common implicated arthropods: bedbugs, mosquitoes, bees, wasps, hornets

PATHOPHYSIOLOGY

- Acute reaction results from mechanical or toxin-mediated tissue trauma.
- Delayed hypersensitivity reaction to antigens in injected protein or saliva of the insect.

CLINICAL FEATURES

- Wide spectrum of lesions depending on involved arthropod.
- Intensely pruritic solitary or multiple urticarial papules.
- Excoriated lesions that are crusted and purulent may represent. secondary infection (most commonly with *S. aureus* or group A *Streptococcus*).

SPECIAL STUDIES

- Commercial venom kits are available for allergy skin testing.
- Serology to investigate systemic infection.

CLINICAL VARIANTS

- None

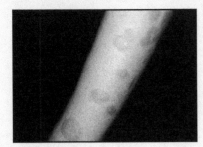

EPIDEMIOLOGY

- Most commonly implicated drugs are
  - Antimicrobials tetracycline
  - NSAIDS
  - Salicylates
  - Phenolphthalein

PATHOPHYSIOLOGY

- The drug in the circulation may act as a hapten and bind to protein components or receptors in the cells of the lower epidermis.
- Both T and B lymphocytes are subsequently stimulated, producing lymphokines and antibodies that could eventually cause inflammation and damage to cells in the basal cell layer.

CLINICAL FEATURES

- Usually appears as a solitary, round or oval, pruritic erythematous macule that subsequently evolves into an edematous plaque with or without vesicles or bullae.
- Residual hyperpigmentation can vary in color from brown to violet-brown or black.

CLINICAL VARIANTS

- Multiple variants have been described (pigmenting, generalized or multiple, linear, wandering, nonpigmenting, bullous, eczematous, urticarial, erythema dyschromicum perstans–like, psoriasiform, and mucosal FDE).

FIXED DRUG ERUPTION

Fixed drug eruption (FDE) is a variant of drug-induced dermatoses with characteristic recurrence at the same site of the skin or mucus membranes. Although a single drug is usually responsible for FDE, there are patients in whom FDE develops following the ingestion of multiple drugs.

HISTOLOGICAL FEATURES

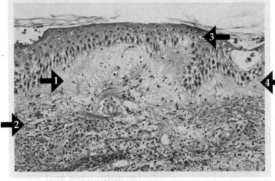

1. Dermal edema
2. Superficial perivascular lymphocytic infiltrate
3. Dyskeratotic keratinocytes
4. Interface vacuolar change

1. Perivascular lymphocytic infiltrate
2. Eosinophils

Other features:
- Normal stratum corneum
- Dermal melanophages

HISTOLOGICAL DIFFERENTIAL

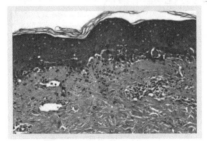

ERYTHEMA MULTIFORME

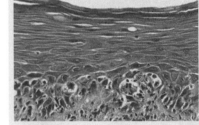

ACUTE GRAFT-VERSUS-HOST DISEASE

- Necrotic keratinocytes found in both
- Less likely to have eosinophils
- Interface dermatitis
- Has only superficial perivascular infiltrate

- Necrotic keratinocytes found in both
- Satellite cell necrosis
- Prominent involvement of follicles
- A sparse superficial perivascular infiltrate
- Correlate clinically

GOOD THINGS TO KNOW

- FDE characteristically recurs at the same site or sites, and with each exposure the number of sites may increase.
- The pigmentation in a given lesion is intensified with each recurrence of FDE.

VASCULITIS

- LEUKOCYTOCLASTIC VASCULITIS
- VASO-OCCLUSIVE VASCULITIS

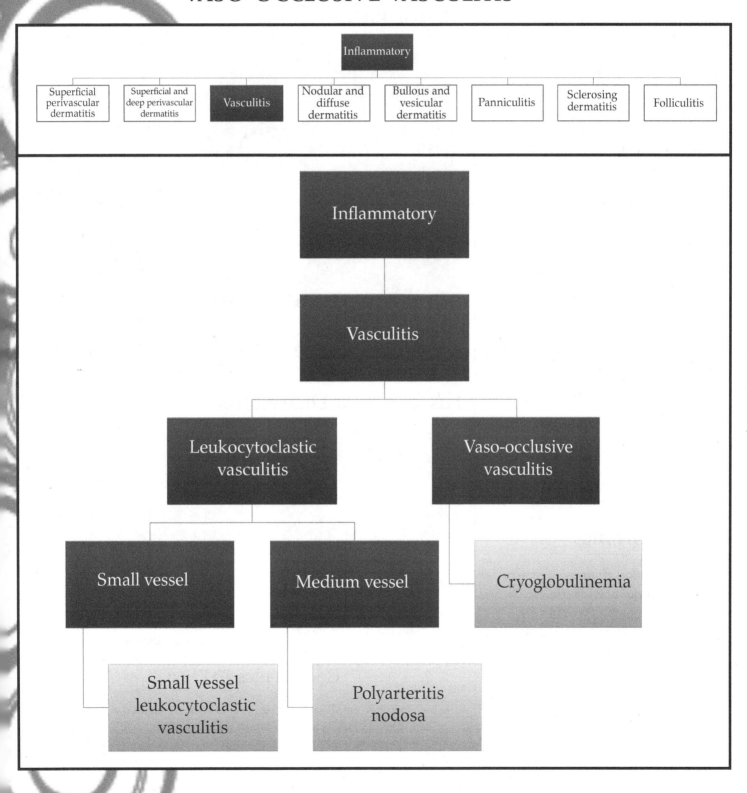

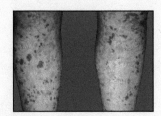

EPIDEMIOLOGY

- More common in adults
- Seen in both males and females

PATHOPHYSIOLOGY

- Many disease processes are characterized with a small vessel neutrophilic vasculitis.
- Multiple etiologies: infectious, immune-mediated, antineutrophil antibody-associated or idiopathic causes.
- Small dermal vessels, particularly the postcapillary venules, are involved.

CLINICAL FEATURES

- Presentation depends on extent of vascular involvement.
  o Most common: palpable purpura located primarily on distal lower extremities.
- Superficial involvement: erythematous and purpuric maculopapules.
- Deeper involvement: infarcts/necrosis and hemorrhagic bullae.

SPECIAL STUDIES

- Microbiological cultures, organism stains, immunofluorescence, or serologic studies to determine the underlying pathological mechanism causing the vasculitis

CLINICAL VARIANTS

- None

SMALL-VESSEL LEUKOCYTOCLASTIC VASCULITIS

Small-vessel leukocytoclastic vasculitis is an inflammatory process involving small vessels in the skin and is associated with a predominantly neutrophilic infiltrate. The differential diagnosis is broad and includes infectious causes to immunologic mediated etiologies.

HISTOLOGICAL FEATURES

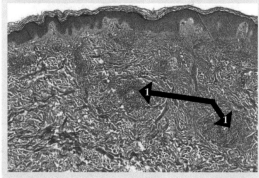

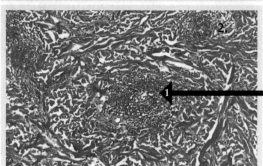

1. **Dense perivascular neutrophilic infiltrate**

1. **Vessel wall invaded by leukocytoclastic neutrophils**

Other features:
- **Dermal vascular damage:**
  - **endothelial cell swelling**
  - **eosinophilic fibrin deposits within vessel walls**
  - **red blood cell extravasation**
- **neutrophilic inflammatory infiltrate predominately involving post capillary venules**
- **Neutrophilic nuclei fragmentation (leukocytoclasis)**

HISTOLOGICAL DIFFERENTIAL

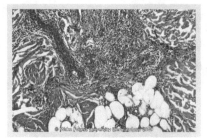

SEPTIC VASCULITIS
(E.G., CHRONIC GONOCOCCEMIA)

- Thrombi present more commonly.
- Arterioles may also be affected.

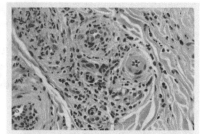

ERYTHEMA ELEVATUM DIUTINUM

- Early lesions show a nonspecific leukocytoclastic vasculitis.
- Fibrinoid deposits in capillaries.
- Fibrosis in late lesions.

GOOD THINGS TO KNOW

- Neutrophilic small-vessel vasculitis is seen in many disease processes, such as Henoch–Schoenlein purpura, cryoglobulinemia, Wegner's granulomatosis, rickettsial infection, and polyarteritis nodosa.

Polyarteritis Nodosa

Polyarteritis nodosa (PAN) is a systemic non-infectious necrotizing disease of small-to-medium-sized arteries. It often presents with cutaneus nodules, neuropathies, myalgias, renal dysfunction, GI involvement, and cardiac abnormalities.

Histological Features

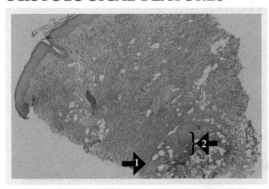

1. **Dermis-subcutis junction**
2. **Involvement of small-medium size arteries**

1. **Inflammatory infiltrate surrounding vessels**
2. **Fibrin deposition and destruction of arterial wall**

• Involves small-to-medium-sized vessels in the dermis and subcutis
• Acute
  - Fibrinoid necrosis of arterial wall
  - Inflammatory infiltrate within and around vessels composed of leukocytoclastic neutrophils and occasional eosinophils
  - Dysmorphic and eosinophilic elastic lamina
• Chronic
  - Subacute infiltrate composed of lymphocytes, histiocytes, and plasma cells
  - Intimal proliferation and thrombosis
  - Fibrinous scarring of vessel wall
  - Necrosis and ulceration

Histological Differential

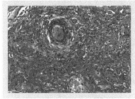

Wegener's Granulomatosis
• Necrotizing small vessel vasculitis
• Palisading granulomatous inflammation
• Suppurative necrosis
• C-ANCA positive

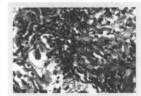

Churg–Strauss Syndrome
• Leukocytoclastic vasculitis
• Eosinophilic granulomatous vasculitis of mid-sized vessels
• Correlate clinically (associated with asthma)

Good Things To Know

• Hepatitis B virus infection is the etiologic trigger in approximately 7% of patients with PAN.

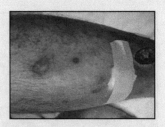

Epidemiology
• Prevalence: 6.3 per 100,000.
• Mean age of onset is 45 years.
• More commonly affects males (M:F, 2.5:1).

Pathophysiology
• Unknown etiology.
• Leukocytoclastic necrotizing vasculitis of the small-to-medium-sized arteries.
• Immune complex and complement deposits trigger recruitment of neutrophils.
• Some studies show macrophage and CD4+ T cell involvement as well.

Clinical Features
• Various cutaneous lesions may be present: subcutaneous nodules, purpura, livedo reticularis, or necrosis and gangrene secondary to ischemia.
• Associated with fever, myalgias, weight loss, and malaise.
• Multisystem: kidney, cardiac, gastrointestinal, and neurological involvement.

Special Studies
• Enzyme linked immunoabsorbent assay (ELISA) and indirect immunofluorescence (DIF) do not detect autoantibodies (ex. ANCA).

Clinical Variants

• "Classic" systemic PAN
• Cutaneous PAN
  - Limited cutaneous disease that may involve the nerves

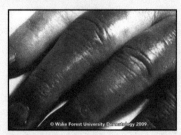

EPIDEMIOLOGY

• Incidence rates vary with the population studied.

PATHOPHYSIOLOGY

• Circulating cryoglobulins precipitate when the skin is cooled and cause hyperviscosity and thrombotic occlusion of the superficial dermal vasculature.
  o Type I: monoclonal immunoglobulins (IgG, IgM, IgA); associated with lympho and myeloproliferative disorders.
  o Type II: mixed immune complexes, monoclonal and polyclonal components; most common is IgG-IgM combination.
  o Type III: polyclonal immunoglobulins; associated with connective tissue disorders and some infections (hepatitis B).

CLINICAL FEATURES

• Various presentations on cold-exposed sites: Raynaud's phenomenon, retiform purpura, acral hemmorhagic necrosis and gangrene of distal extremities, etc.

SPECIAL STUDIES

• To detect cryoglobulins, a blood sample is drawn into a warmed syringe; after removing the erythrocytes the plasma is cooled and centrifuged to isolate the cryoprecipitate.

CLINICAL VARIANTS

• None

CRYOGLOBULINEMIA

Cryoglobulinemia is a small vessel vasculitis associated with deposited paraproteins. There are three subtypes: type I involves monoclonal globulins, and types II and III are known as mixed cryoglobulinemias.

HISTOLOGICAL FEATURES

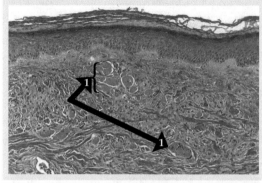

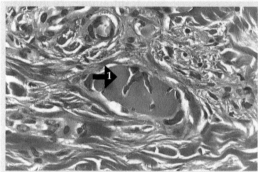

1. **Thrombosed dermal vasculature**

1. **PAS-positive cryoprecipitate occluding vessel**

• Epidermis may be normal, necrotic, or ulcerated.
• Cryoprecipitate in superficial dermal blood vessels occlude lumen and stain bright red with periodic acid-Schiff stain (PAS).
• Extravasated erythrocytes.

• Leukocytoclastic vasculitis is seen in mixed cryoglobulinemias (types II and III).
• PAS-positive vascular precipitates are seen less often in the mixed subtypes.

HISTOLOGICAL DIFFERENTIAL

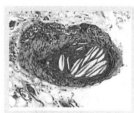

CUTANEOUS CHOLESTEROL EMBOLISM

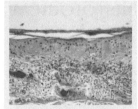

DISSEMINATED INTRAVAS-CULAR COAGULATION

GOOD THINGS TO KNOW

• Mixed cryoglobulinemia cannot be distinguished histologically from other forms of leukocytoclastic vasculitides.

• Needle-shaped cholesterol clefts within vessel lumen
• Foreign-body granuloma reaction

• Fibrin deposits stain less intensely with PAS.
• Later stages have more widespread infiltrates and tissue necrosis.

NODULAR AND DIFFUSE DERMATITIS
• NODULAR (GRANULOMATOUS) DERMATITIS

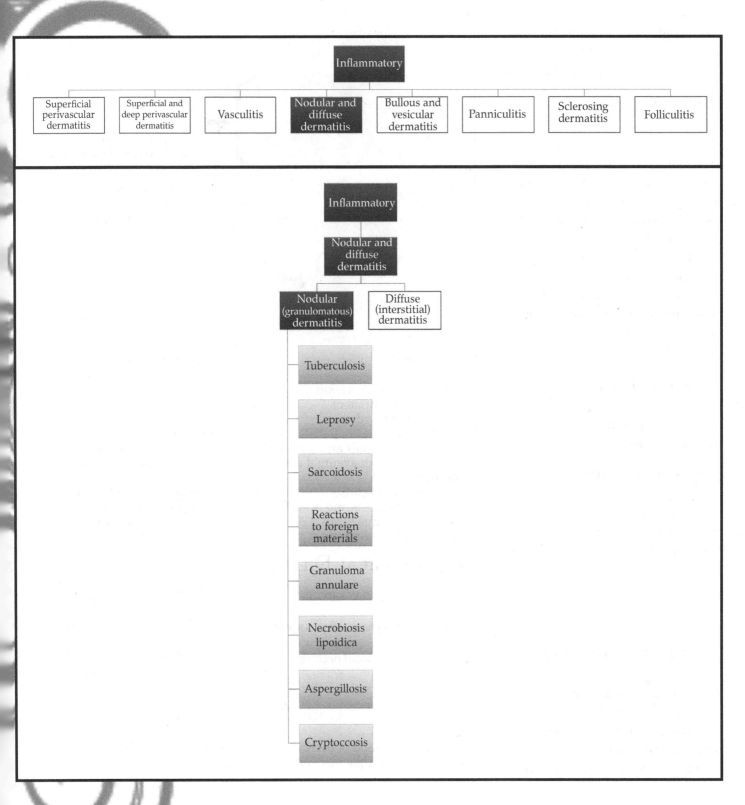

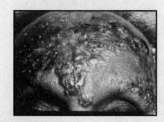

EPIDEMIOLOGY

• In the U.S., rates of TB have declined.
• Although 1 of 3 individuals world-wide is infected with *M. tuberculosis*, the incidence of cutaneous TB is low.

PATHOPHYSIOLOGY

• Mycobacterial bacilli induce an acute nonspecific inflammation during which bacilli multiply. Macrophages phagocytose organisms, and kill the bacilli once they are activated by T cells. Activated macrophages transform to epithelioid cells or fuse to form giant cells.
• The magnitude and type of inflammatory response are highly dependent on the cell-mediated immune status of the host.

CLINICAL FEATURES

• Presentation is dependent on the type of cutaneous TB.

SPECIAL STUDIES

• Acid fast stains (like Ziehl–Neelsen) reveal pink bacilli.
• PCR on paraffin sections to detect mycobacterial DNA.

CLINICAL VARIANTS

• Tuberculous chancre, tuberculosis verrucosa cutis, lupus vulgaris, scrofuloderma, orificial tuberculosis, acute miliary tuberculosis, tuberculous gumma

TUBERCULOSIS

Tuberculosis (TB) is an infection caused by *Mycobacterium tuberculosis* and is the most common cause of infectious disease–related mortality worldwide. There are many forms of systemic TB and cutaneous TB.

HISTOLOGICAL FEATURES

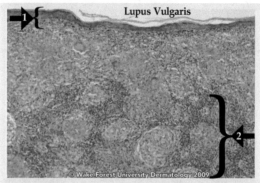

Lupus Vulgaris

1. Epidermal atrophy
2. Tuberculoid granulomas

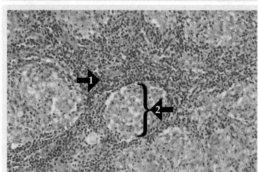

1. Dense lymphocytic infiltrate
2. Minimal caseation

• Primary TB (tuberculous chancre)
  - epidermal ulceration
  - mixed infiltrate of macrophages and many neutrophils
  - epithelioid cells and giant cell granulomas with eventual caseous necrosis
• TB verrucosa cutis:
  - hyperkeratosis and acanthosis
  - subepidermal acute inflammatory infiltrate

  - dermal granulomas with necrosis
• Lupus vulgaris
  - epidermal atrophy or hyperplasia
  - tuberculoid granulomas with scant to no caseating necrosis
  - numerous Langhans-type giant cells
  - pronounced lymphocytic infiltrate in upper dermis; may extend to subcutaneous layer

HISTOLOGICAL DIFFERENTIAL

SARCOIDOSIS

• Less lymphocytic reaction surrounding granulomas
• Presence of fibrinoid necrosis

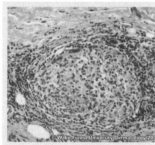

GOOD THINGS TO KNOW

• The likelihood of detecting bacilli or culturing mycobacteria is dependent on the form of cutaneous TB.

Leprosy (Hansen's disease)

Leprosy (Hansen's disease) is a chronic infectious disease caused by *Mycobacterium leprae*. There are two major forms of this disease: tuberculoid and lepromatous.

Histological Features

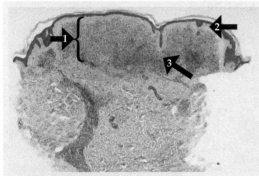

1. **Diffuse infiltrate by foamy macrophages**
2. **Grenz zone**
3. **No granuloma formation**

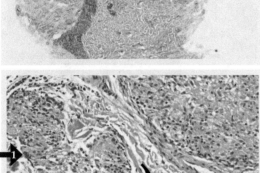

1. Tuberculoid leprosy
2. Granuloma formation

- Lepromatous
  - grenz zone (normal zone of collagen separates the epidermis from diffuse dermal infiltrate)
  - no granuloma formation
  - numerous globi (foamy macrophages filled with *M. leprae*)
- Tuberculoid
  - no grenz zone
  - large epitheloid granulomas
  - rare/absent acid fast bacilli (AFB)

Histological Differential

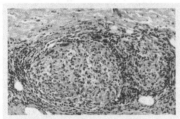

Sarcoidosis
- Presence of non-caseating granulomas
- No granulomas in dermal nerves
- No AFB

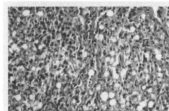

Cutaneous Leishmaniasis
- Inflammatory cell infiltrate composed of macrophages with amastigotes expand the dermal papilla.
- Presence of Leishman–Donovan bodies within the macrophages.

Good Things To Know

- Erythema nodosum leprosum, an immune-mediated reaction, may occur and severe cases may be treated with thalidomide.

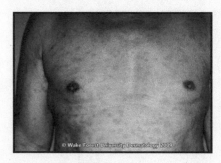

Epidemiology

- About 100 new cases every year in the U.S. – most of which are immigrants from endemic areas such as Southeast Asia and Latin America.
- Predisposing factors: sex, socio-economic status, and immune function.

Pathophysiology

- Transmitted via aerosols and contact.
- Tuberculoid leprosy occurs with an intact cell-mediated response to infection.
- Lepromatous subtype seen in anergic response.
- A range of intermediate states between these two clinical manifestations exist.

Clinical Features

- Tuberculoid: hypopigmented macules and variable loss of sensation
- Lepromatous: dull red papules and nodules; lion-like facial features; minimal sensory involvement

Special Studies

- Lepromin testing, acid fast stain, serology, reverse transcriptase PCR

Clinical Variants

- Early, Indeterminate Leprosy
- Lepromatous Leprosy
- Histoid Leprosy
- Borderline Lepromatous Leprosy
- Borderline Tuberculoid Leprosy
- Tuberculoid Leprosy

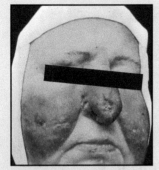

EPIDEMIOLOGY

• In the US, more common in African Americans than Caucasians.

• Onset: commonly <40 years old.

• Cutaneous lesions present most often at the onset of disease, although they can occur at any stage.

PATHOPHYSIOLOGY

• Unknown underlying etiology, involves a macrophage/Th1 cell mediated non-caseating.

granulomatous inflammatory process

• Genetic factors may play a role. Familial cases seen in 15% of patients; MHC genes on short arm of chromosome 6 have been implicated.

CLINICAL FEATURES

• Erythema nodosum is the most common nonspecific cutaneous lesion from sarcoidosis.

• Lesions range from smooth violaceous nodules located on the nose/cheeks/earlobes (lupus pernio) to diffuse maculopapules or brown-purple indurated papules or nodules with an annular/serpiginous pattern

SPECIAL STUDIES

• Serum angiotensin converting enzymes (ACE) are elevated.

• Hypergammaglobulinemia and hypercalcemia are often present.

CLINICAL VARIANTS

• None

SARCOIDOSIS

Sarcoidosis is a multisystemic idiopathic disease characterized by noncaseating granulomas, most commonly affecting the lungs and hilar lymph nodes. Cutaneous lesions are present in 25–35% of cases.

HISTOLOGICAL FEATURES

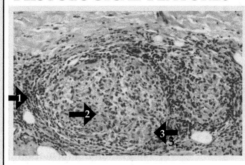

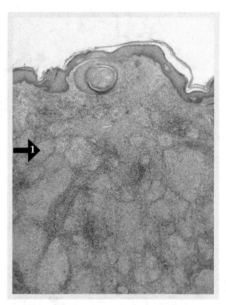

1. **Well-formed granuolma**
2. **No central necrosis**
3. **Epitheloid macrophages**

1. **"Naked" granulomas, composed of epitheliod cells and multinucleated giant cells with none to few lymphocytes**

• Asteroid bodies (stellate inclusions within giant cells), Schaumann bodies (inclusions of calcium and protein in the cytoplasm of giant cells), and Hamazaki–Wesenberg bodies are nonspecific features but may be present.

• If chronic, granulomas may be surrounded by a fibrous rim or replaced by a hyaline fibrous scar.

HISTOLOGICAL DIFFERENTIAL

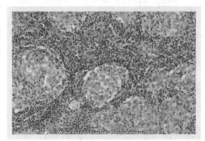

LUPUS VULGARIS

FOREIGN BODY GRANULOMAS

• The infiltrate is located more toward the epidermis.

• Characterized by marked inflammatory infiltrate surrounding the granulomas.

• Granulomas have more central necrosis.

• Presence of foreign material, ex. doubly refractile material such as silica, under polariscopic examination.

• Giant cell nuclei can be of foreign-body origin, arranged in a haphazard array.

• Infiltration of lymphocytes, neutrophils, and plasma cells.

GOOD THINGS TO KNOW

• Can be localized to scars

REACTION TO FOREIGN MATERIALS

Endogenous or exogenous deposits can produce a granulomatous body reaction in the dermis, where it is perceived as foreign material.

HISTOLOGICAL FEATURES

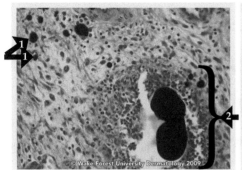

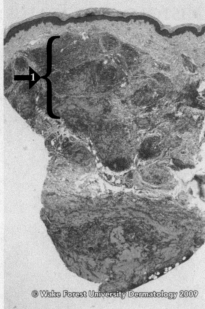

1. Implanted mercury pigment
2. Granuloma formation surrounding the foreign material

1. Granulomatous infiltrate surrounding injected bovine collagen

Other features:
- Giant cells may be foreign body type: multiple nuclei arranged in a haphazard array.
- Variable inflammatory infiltrate, including lymphocytes, plasma cells, and neutrophils.
- "Knife-marks" – nodular collections of epithelioid histiocytes.
- An allergic reaction may show a sarcoidal or tuberculoid pattern of epithelioid cells with or without giant cells.

HISTOLOGICAL DIFFERENTIAL

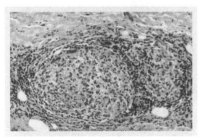

SARCOIDOSIS

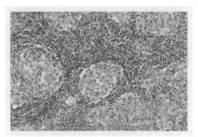

TUBERCULOSIS

- Absence of foreign material
- Diffuse noncaseating granulomatous infiltration in the dermis
- No giant cells of foreign origin

- Absence of foreign material
- May have minimal caseation
- Tuberculoid granulomas

GOOD THINGS TO KNOW

- Most common cause of a foreign body granuloma is a follicular cyst or rupture of a hair follicle.

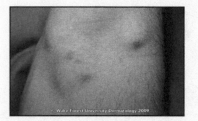

EPIDEMIOLOGY
- Endogenous materials:
  - Sodium urate crystals in gout
  - Keratinous material (ex. cornified cells or hair without an epithelial coat)
- Exogenous materials:
  - Sutures
  - Tattoo pigments
  - Silica, berylliosis
  - Mercury
  - Collagen implants
  - Injectable corticosteroids

PATHOPHYSIOLOGY
- Foreign material can be accidently implanted and introduced in the dermis (ex. splinter).
- Inert materials that are too large to be phagocytosed by macrophages and neutrophils that reside in the dermis cause a granulomatous reaction.
- Individuals sensitized to the particular substance may also mount an allergic response to the materials.

CLINICAL FEATURES
- Presentation is dependent on the foreign material, location, and how it was introduced into the dermis.
- Usually presents as a firm erythematous palpable nodule clearly demarcated from the surrounding normal skin.

SPECIAL STUDIES
- Polariscopic examination can reveal foreign substance, ex. a doubly refractile material like silica.

CLINICAL VARIANTS
- None

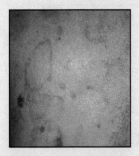

EPIDEMIOLOGY

- More common in females
- Most commonly seen in childhood through early adulthood
- Unknown etiology

PATHOPHYSIOLOGY

- Suspected that a cell-mediated immune response and a delayed hypersensitivity reaction occur following trauma, viral infections, or malignancy. These responses lead to the degeneration of collagen and macrophage invasion in the affected tissue(s).

CLINICAL FEATURES

- Usually asymptomatic.
- Lesions can be flesh-colored, tan, erythematous or violaceous
- Most commonly presents as dermal papules and annular plaques with central clearing localized on the hands and feet, or can be generalized.
- Subcutaneous GA: nodules on scalp or palmoplantar surfaces.
- Perforating GA: lesions have central ulceration.

SPECIAL STUDIES

- None

CLINICAL VARIANTS

- Subcutaneous GA
- Perforating GA

GRANULOMA ANNULARE

Granuloma annulare (GA) is an idiopathic palisading granulomatous disease that typically presents with annular lesions on the hands and feet but can also present in a generalized pattern. Less common forms of GA include subcutaneous GA and perforating GA.

HISTOLOGICAL FEATURES

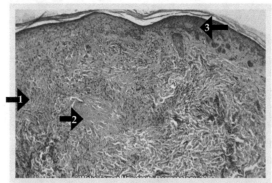

1. Nodular dermatitis
2. Dermal necrobiosis and mucin deposits with surrounding palisaded macrophages and multinucleated giant cell
3. Normal epidermis

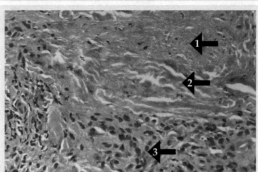

1. Mucin deposits
2. Degenerated collagen
3. Palisading histiocytes

HISTOLOGICAL DIFFERENTIAL

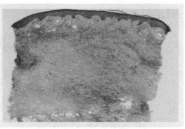

NECROBIOSIS LIPOIDICA
- More extensive involvement, affects subcutaneous tissue
- Degenerative collagen in dermis (necrobiosis)
- Presence of plasma cells
- Lacks central mucin deposition

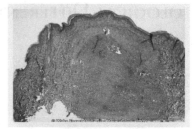

RHEUMATOID NODULE
- Subcutaneous necrobiotic nodule
- More eosinophilic hue
- Clinical diagnosis crucial to accurately distinguish from subcutaneous GA

GOOD THINGS TO KNOW
- GA is often misdiagnosed as tinea corporis.
- There is some association between generalized GA and diabetes mellitus.
- Subcutaneous GA nodules clinically resemble rheumatoid nodules.

NECROBIOSIS LIPOIDICA

Necrobiosis lipoidica (NL) is a rare, chronic, noninfectious granulomatous disease of connective tissue degeneration oftentimes presenting as yellow-brown plaques on the shins of diabetics.

HISTOLOGICAL FEATURES

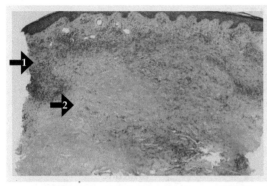

1. Palisading granulomas surrounding layered, degenerated collagen (necrobiosis) in the dermis often extending into the subcutaneous tissue
2. Necrobiosis

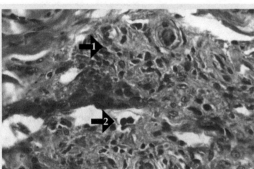

1. Perivascular infiltrate
2. Plasma cells

Other features:
• Normal or atrophic epidermis, possibly with ulceration
• Mixed inflammatory infiltrate, including plasma cells arranged parallel to the epidermis surrounded by horizontally oriented necrobiosis and in perivascular regions

HISTOLOGICAL DIFFERENTIAL

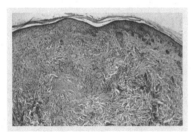

GRANULOMA ANNULARE

• Mucin in necrobiotic areas
• Round/focal palisades
• Lack of plasma cells

RHEUMATOID NODULE

• More eosinophilic hue
• Fibrin located deep in dermis
• Subcutaneous necrobiotic palisades

GOOD THINGS TO KNOW

• Rare reports of squamous cell carcinomas arising in areas of NL

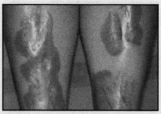

EPIDEMIOLOGY

• Predisposing factors: Type I diabetes mellitus (necrobiosis lipoidica diabeticorum; prevalence is 3/1000), less frequently Type II diabetes mellitus, Crohn's disease, ulcerative colitis; granuloma annulare, sarcoidosis.
• Average age of onset is 30–40 years, more often seen in females (F:M, 3:1).

PATHOPHYSIOLOGY

• Unknown etiology, but hypothesized to be secondary to either diabetic microangiopathy or antibody-mediated vasculitis
• Collagen degeneration with surrounding noninfectious granulomatous inflammation and thickened blood vessel walls

CLINICAL FEATURES

• Red patches that enlarge to yellow-brown plaques with shiny, central atrophy and telangiectasias.
• Most commonly located on pretibial regions, less frequently on face, scalp, trunk, and upper extremities; may be unilateral or bilateral.
• Ulcers may be induced by trauma; may be painful or secondarily infected.
• Spontaneous remission with residual scar and atrophy possible.

SPECIAL STUDIES

• In diabetics, DIF would show IgM, IgA, C3, and fibrinogen in blood vessels, resulting in vascular thickening.
• H&E is the stain of choice.

CLINICAL VARIANTS

• None

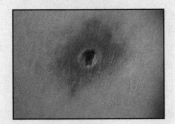

EPIDEMIOLOGY

• *Aspergillus fumigatus* is the most common causative human pathogen.
• Most commonly seen in immuno-compromised patients.
• Risk factors include farming, the use of long-term and/or broad spectrum antibiotics, chronic corticosteroid use, bone marrow suppression/transplantation, burn victims, and long-term hospitalizations.

PATHOPHYSIOLOGY

• The usual portal of entry is inhalation of fungal spores.
• Localized pulmonary disease can result in allergic aspergillosis, fungus balls, or necrotizing pneumonia.
• Immunocompromised states. perpetuate fungal dissemination and invasive disease.
• Cutaneous aspergillosis can arise due to primary inoculation or secondary to disseminated disease.

CLINICAL FEATURES

• Initial cutaneous features include erythematous macular, papular, vesicular or bullous lesions.
• Lesions will later progress into necrotic ulcers with a central eschar surface.
• Also presents with constitutional symptoms including fever, chills, and sweats.

SPECIAL STUDIES

• Gomori methanamine silver staining
• KOH preparation
• Fungal culture

CLINICAL VARIANTS

• None

ASPERGILLOSIS

Aspergillosis is a ubiquitous fungal organism that most commonly infects immunocompromised adults. Cutaneous manifestations are clinically characterized by a necrotic papule with a central eschar surface. Histologically, hyphae are described as having acute-angle branching (approximately 45°) with frequent septations.

HISTOLOGICAL FEATURES

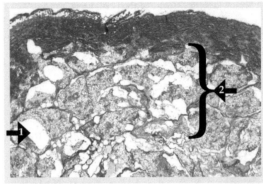

1. Dermal necrosis
2. Scant inflammatory infiltrate

1. Numerous 2–4 μm in diameter hyphae branching at a 45° angle
2. Hyphae with septa

Other features:
• Pseudoepitheliomatous hyperplasia
• Variable granulomatous infiltrate of neutrophils, lymphocytes, giant cells, and histiocytes

HISTOLOGICAL DIFFERENTIAL

MUCORMYCOSIS

• Absence of septa.
• Broad hypae that branch at irregular intervals in 90° angles.
• Fungal organisms may be visible within vessels.

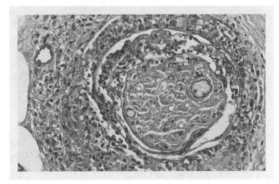

GOOD THINGS TO KNOW

• Definitive diagnosis requires a fungal culture.

CRYPTOCOCCOSIS

Cryptococcosis is an infection caused by the encapsulated yeast, *Cryptococcus neoformans*. It is typically acquired from the inhalation of spores in bird droppings (especially pigeon) and can then disseminate from the lungs to the CNS, bones, and skin.

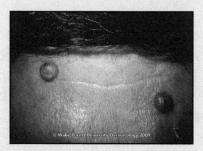

HISTOLOGICAL FEATURES

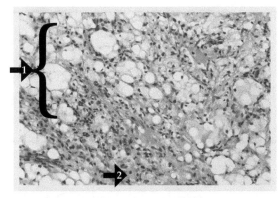

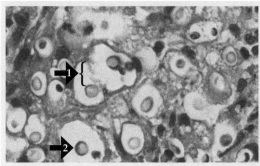

1. H&E stains visualize spores but not the surrounding capsules.
2. Mixed inflammatory infiltrate.

∞∞∞∞∞∞∞∞∞∞∞∞∞∞∞∞∞∞∞∞∞∞∞∞

1. Thick capsule
2. Aggregates of encapsulated narrow based, unequal budding yeasts, ranging from 2–15µm

Other features:
• Either or a combined pattern of
  - Granulomatous pattern: infiltrate of lymphocytes, histiocytes, multinucleated giant cells, and neutrophils in the dermis; small number of organisms present without a capsule.
  - Gelatinous pattern: large number of spores, little inflammation.

HISTOLOGICAL DIFFERENTIAL

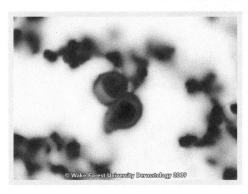

BLASTOMYCOSIS

• Broad-based budding yeast
• Does not stain black with Fontana–Masson stain

EPIDEMIOLOGY

• Occurs most commonly in immunocompromised adults.
• More common in men (M:F, 2:1).
• 90% of cases are localized to the lungs.

PATHOPHYSIOLOGY

• Causes a primary lung infection through the inhalation of spores.
• Can then disseminate to the CNS, bone, and skin, causing secondary cutaneous cryptococcosis.
• Primary cutaneous cryptococcosis rarely occurs via direct inoculation.
• The yeast has a special affinity for the CNS and is the most common cause of mycotic meningitis.

CLINICAL FEATURES

• Variable cutaneous manifestations
  o Presents as a papulonodular eruption, cellulitis, abscess, pustule or ulcer

SPECIAL STUDIES

• India ink, Alcian blue with PAS stain, mucicarmine to stain the capsule
• Fontana–Masson stain to highlight the melanin contained in the cell wall
• Latex agglutination test to detect the cryptococcal capsular polysaccharide antigen

CLINICAL VARIANTS

• None

GOOD THINGS TO KNOW

• Yeasts have a wider capsule when there is less inflammation, such as in a severely immunocompromised patient.

• DIFFUSE (INTERSTITIAL) DERMATITIS

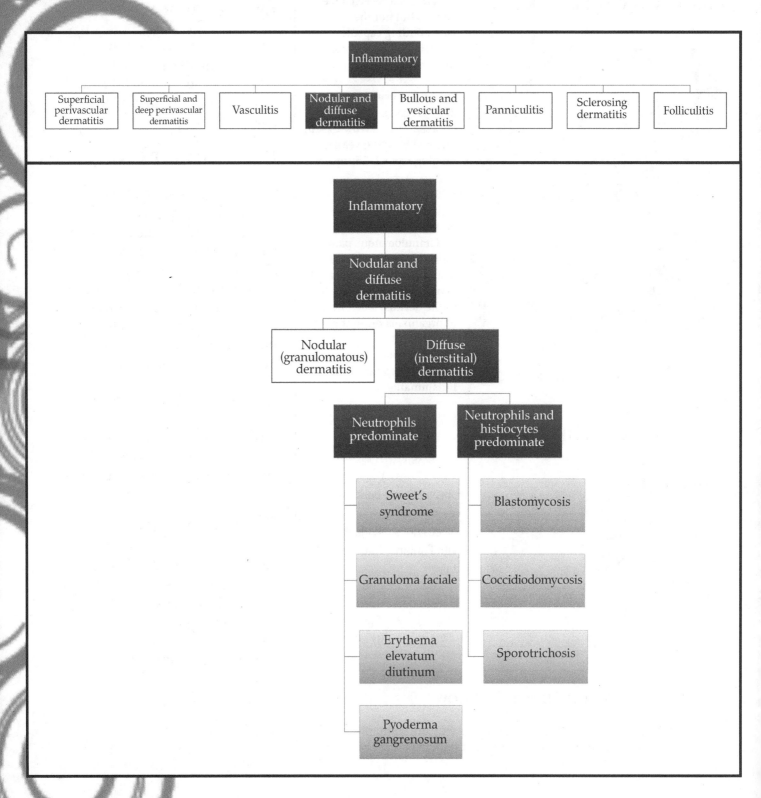

Sweet's Syndrome

Sweet's syndrome, or acute febrile neutrophilic dermatosis, is an idiopathic disease characterized by the typical eruption of erythematous plaques infiltrated by neutrophils.

Histological Features

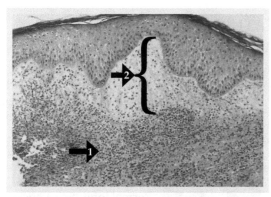

1. **Papillary dermal edema**
2. **Dense perivascular neutrophilic infiltrate in the upper dermis**

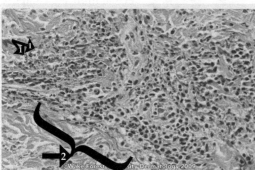

1. **Extravasated erythrocytes**
2. **Neutrophilic infiltrate**

Other features:
- **Neutrophilic leukocytoclasis (nuclear fragmentation).**
- **Vascular changes may be present: erythrocyte extravasation, endothelial swelling, vasodilation.**

Histological Differential

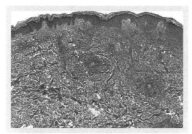

LEUKOCYTOCLASTIC VASCULITIS

- Fibrinoid degeneration of dermal vasculature:
  - endothelial cell swelling
  - eosinophilic fibrin deposits in vessel walls

PYODERMA GANGRENOSUM

- Neutrophilic infiltrate is more extensive and deeper in dermis.
- Infiltrate frequently involves follicular structures.

Good Things To Know

- Sweet's Syndrome has various associations: underlying malignancies, bacterial infections, drugs, autoimmune and collagen vascular diseases, inflammatory bowel disease, or pregnancy.

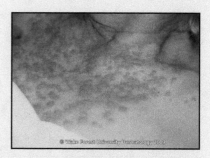

Epidemiology

- Female predominance (4:1, F:M).
- Mean age of onset is 56 years old.
- Classically, upper respiratory tract infection or tonsillitis precedes disease by 1–3 weeks.

Pathophysiology

- Unknown etiology, but may be a hypersensitivity reaction.
- Implicated cytokine dysregulation includes interleukin IL-1, IL-3, IL-6, IL-8, granulocyte colony-stimulating factor (G-CSF), granulocyte-macrophage colony stimulating factor- (GM-CSF), and interferon gamma.

Clinical Features

- Primary features include a cutaneous painful eruption of erythematous papules and plaques that may appear vesiculated due to edema.
- Lesions favor the face, neck, and upper extremities.

Special Studies

- Direct immunofluorescence studies are generally negative.

Clinical Variants

- None

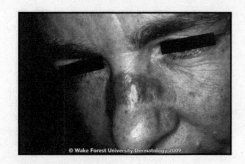

EPIDEMIOLOGY

• Rare disorder that is most commonly seen in healthy middle-aged white males

PATHOPHYSIOLOGY

• Idiopathic etiology.
• Studies suggest it may be associated with sun exposure in a pathway mediated by interleukin-5 and/or gamma-interferon.

CLINICAL FEATURES

• Asymptomatic single or multiple papules, plaques, or nodules, with
  o well-defined borders.
  o color varying from a dull red to dark purple.
  o Soft and smooth texture
• Most commonly found on the face

SPECIAL STUDIES

• None

CLINICAL VARIANTS

• None

GRANULOMA FACIALE

Granuloma faciale (GF) is a chronic skin disorder that presents with cutaneous lesions typically seen on the face. Histologically, GF is characterized by a grenz zone and a polymorphous dermal infiltrate.

HISTOLOGICAL FEATURES

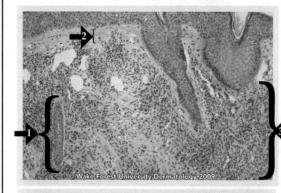

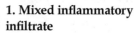

1. Undisrupted hair follicle
2. Zone of normal collagen that separates the epidermis from the dermal infiltrate (grenz zone)
3. Dense polymorphous dermal infiltrate composed of neutrophils, eosinophils, and plasma cells

1. Mixed inflammatory infiltrate
2. Eosinophil
Other features:
• Variable evidence of vascular damage
• Fragmented neutrophilic nuclei (nuclear dust)
• Undisrupted pilosebaceous structures

HISTOLOGICAL DIFFERENTIAL

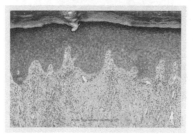

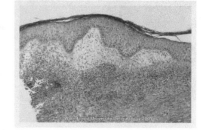

ERYTHEMA ELEVATUM DIUTINUM

• No grenz zone
• Lack of prominent eosino-phils and plasma cells
• Vertically oriented vessels

SWEET'S SYNDROME

• No grenz zone
• Papillary dermal edema
• Vascular changes
• RBC extravasation, endothelial cell swelling

GOOD THINGS TO KNOW

• GF is a misnomer; it is not a granulomatous disorder, but rather a persistent form of leukocytoclastic vasculitis.

ERYTHEMA ELEVATUM DIUTINUM

Erythema elevatum diutinum (EED) is a rare small vessel vasculitis characterized by violaceous papules most commonly on the extensor surfaces of the extremities. Histologic features depend on the stage of disease and range from leukocytoclastic vasculitis to fibrosis.

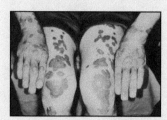

HISTOLOGICAL FEATURES

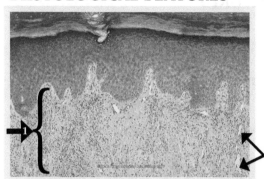

1. Diffuse polymorphous inflammatory infiltrate
2. Vertically oriented vessels in dermis

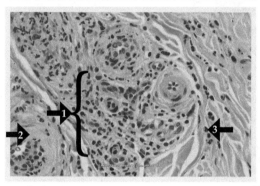

1. Mixed inflammatory infiltrate
2. Fibrous thickening of vasculature
3. Neutrophil

- Early lesions:
  - Nonspecific leukocytoclastic vasculitis
- Mature lesions:
  - Diffuse polymorphous infiltrate, predominance of neutrophils
- Fibrinoid deposits in capillaries
- Vertically oriented vessels
- Late lesions:
  - Extracellular cholesterol clefts
  - Fibrosis and sclerosis

HISTOLOGICAL DIFFERENTIAL

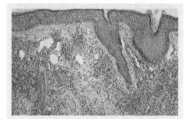

GRANULOMA FACIALE
- Presence of grenz zone
- Predominance of eosinophils and plasma cells in addition to neutrophils
- Clinical localization

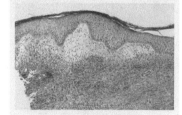

SWEET'S SYNDROME
- Both have neutrophilic leukocytoclasis.
- No fibrosis.
- Correlate clinically.

GOOD THINGS TO KNOW

- Atypical features include bullae, necrotizing granulomas, and neutrophilic microabscesses in the tips of the dermal papillae.

EPIDEMIOLOGY

- Rare, no racial or gender predilection.
- Most common in adults 30–60 years old.
- Associated with
  o Autoimmune diseases (SLE)
  o Inflammatory bowel disease
  o Hematological disorders
  o HIV-infection

PATHOPHYSIOLOGY

- Hypothesized to be secondary to invasion of circulating immune complexes into the dermal perivascular spaces or a hypersensitivity reaction to chronic antigen exposure.
- The resultant complement activation, neutrophilic infiltration, and release of enzymes cause progressive fibrin deposition in and around small dermal vessels.

CLINICAL FEATURES

- Symmetrical distribution of violaceous, red–brown or yellowish papules, plaques or nodules on the extensor surfaces of the hands and knees
- Asymptomatic to painful or pruritic lesions

SPECIAL STUDIES

- None

CLINICAL VARIANTS

- None

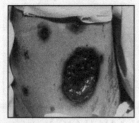

EPIDEMIOLOGY

- More common in females between 20–50 years old
- Associated with systemic diseases:
  - inflammatory bowel disease
  - myeloproliferative disorders
  - arthritis

PATHOPHYSIOLOGY

- Underlying etiology is unknown.
- Classified under neutrophilic dermatosis due to the dense neutrophilic infiltrates found in the skin.
- Humoral, cell-mediated immunity, neutrophilic and monocytic dysfunction have been implicated.
- May have an underlying autoimmune component.

CLINICAL FEATURES

- Clinical course may be acute and rapidly progressive or chronic with spontaneous resolution.
- Painful erythematous papulopustules and nodules commonly found on the lower extremities.
- Can develop central ulceration and necrosis with a purulent base and a characteristic ragged, undermined gunmetal-colored border.
- Isolated or multiple lesions occur usually <3 cm in diameter but may coalesce to form large, rapidly expanding lesions.

SPECIAL STUDIES

- Infectious etiologies must be ruled out by cultures and special stains.

CLINICAL VARIANTS

- Ulcerative PG
- Pustular PG
- Vegetative PG

PYODERMA GANGRENOSUM

Pyoderma gangrenosum (PG) is a rare idiopathic neutrophilic dermatosis. It is a severely debilitating skin disease that is characterized by neutrophilic infiltration and tissue destruction.

HISTOLOGICAL FEATURES

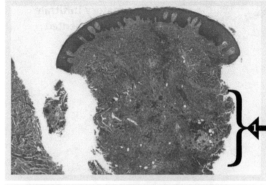

1. Mixed inflammatory infiltrate with a predominance of neutrophils extending deep within the dermis, can also involve follicular structures

1. Neutrophils and lymphocytes surrounding blood vessels
2. Dense inflammatory infiltrate

Other features:
- Ulceration and necrosis
- Acanthosis and spongiosis at the periphery of an ulcer

HISTOLOGICAL DIFFERENTIAL

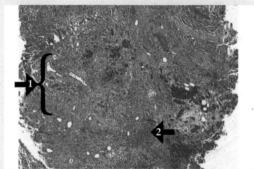
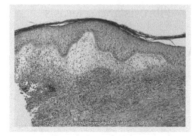

SWEET'S SYNDROME	LEUKOCYTOCLASTIC VASCULITIS
- Less extensive dermal infiltrate - Neutrophilic infiltrate localized more in the papillary dermis - Papillary dermal edema	- Predominantly lymphocytic infiltrate - Fibrinoid degeneration of dermal vasculature

GOOD THINGS TO KNOW

- Histopathological findings are quite variable, and dependent on what stage and where the lesion is biopsied.

Blastomycosis

Blastomycosis is a fungal infection caused by the thermally dimorphic fungus *Blastomyces dermatitidis*. Most often it causes pulmonary infection, but the skin is the most common extrapulmonary site of infection with about 20–40% of patients showing cutaneous involvement.

Histological Features

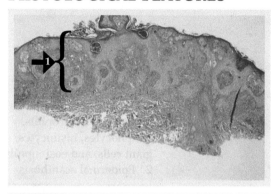

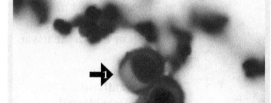

1. **Pseudoepitheliomatous hyperplasia with micro-abcesses**

1. **Thick-walled spores, 5–15 μm in diameter**

Other features:
- **Granulomatous reaction in the dermis of lymphocytes, neutrophils, and giant cells.**
- **Broad-based budding yeasts are demonstrated in the dermis or in giant cells using PAS stains.**

Histological Differential

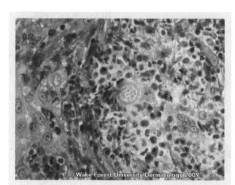

COCCIDIOIDOMYCOSIS

- Larger spores (up to 80 μm) containing numerous endospores

Good Things To Know

- Visualizing the organism is important to differentiate from squamous cell carcinoma.

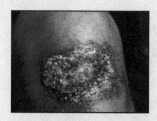

Epidemiology

- Endemic in the Mississippi and Ohio River Valleys
- Incidence of 1:100,000 in Mississippi, Arkansas, Wisconsin, and Kentucky
- More common in immunocompromised adults

Pathophysiology

- Conidia are inhaled causing a primary pulmonary infection.
- In cutaneous blastomycosis, conidia disseminate via the blood or lymphatics to the skin.
- Rarely, cutaneous blastomyosis can result from direct inoculation into the skin from a dog bite or accidental lab inoculation.

Clinical Features

- Approximately 50% of infected people are asymptomatic.
- Lesions are most commonly found on the face, neck, and extremities.
- Early skin lesions are asymptomatic or are mildly tender papules or nodules.
- Later lesions either ulcerate or form plaques with elevated verrucous borders, crust and drainage

Special Studies

- PAS stain for yeast forms; Gomori's methenamine silver (GMS) and Papanicolaou stains will also stain yeast.

Clinical Variants

- None

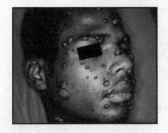

EPIDEMIOLOGY

• In the US, it is endemic in the southwestern states
• Populations at risk: farmers, construction workers, immunocompromised, and people with significant outdoor exposure

PATHOPHYSIOLOGY

• Inhaled arthrospores change morphology into spherules in the lungs, and eventually rupture and disseminate into the blood.
• Most people clear the infection via Th1 mediated immunity.
• Direct inoculation into the skin causes primary cutaneous infections.

CLINICAL FEATURES

• "Classic" finding in disseminated infection: verrucous papule on the nasolabial fold.
• Primary pulmonary infection can be associated with erythema nodosum, erythema multiforme, Sweet's syndrome, or a generalized morbilliform rash.
• Ulcerated nodules with lymphadenopathy at sites of primary cutaneous infection.

SPECIAL STUDIES

• Gomori's methenamine silver (GMS) and PAS stain spherules

CLINICAL VARIANTS

• None

COCCIDIOIDOMYCOSIS

Coccidioidomycosis is a fungal infection caused by the soil-inhabiting dimorphic fungus *Coccidioides immitis*. Infection can present in three forms: primary cutaneous, pulmonary, and systemic.

HISTOLOGICAL FEATURES

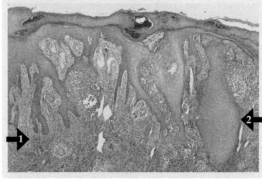

1. Diffuse granulomatous infiltrate of neutrophils, lymphocytes, histiocytes, giant cells, and eosinophils
2. Epidermal acanthosis

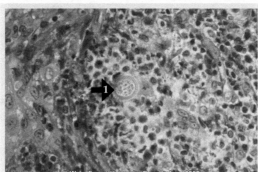

1. Spherule containing numerous endospores measuring 1–4 μm may be present within giant cells or free in the tissue.

Other features:
• Acanthosis
• Intraepidermal microabcesses

HISTOLOGICAL DIFFERENTIAL

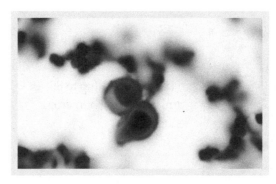

BLASTOMYCOSIS

• Differentiate via culture or histopathological analysis of the organism structure
• Broad-based budding yeasts are smaller in size

GOOD THINGS TO KNOW

• None

Sporotrichosis

Sporotrichosis is an infection caused by the dimorphic fungus *Sporothrix schenckii*. The disease can manifest as a chronic cutaneous or subcutaneous infection, but can rarely become systemic secondary to hematogenous spread. Cutaneous infections are categorized as fixed cutaneous or lymphocutaneous.

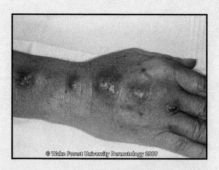

Histological Features

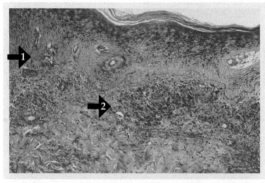

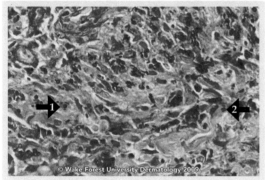

1. Pseudoepitheliomatous epidermal hyperplasia
2. Inflammatory infiltrate in the dermis

◇◇◇◇◇◇◇◇◇◇◇◇◇◇◇◇◇◇◇◇◇◇◇◇◇◇◇◇◇◇

1. Budding round spore of *S. schenckii*
2. Organisms may appear as round-oval spores measuring 4–6 μm in diameter or cigar-shaped bodies.

Other features:
• Early lesions show a nonspecific inflammatory infiltrate of predominately histiocytes and neutrophils, lymphoid cells, and plasma cells in the dermis with scattered granulomas.
• Later subcutaneous nodules form suppurative granulomas surrounded by zones of epithelioid macrophages and lymphocytes which may coalesce to form a large abscess.

Histological Differential

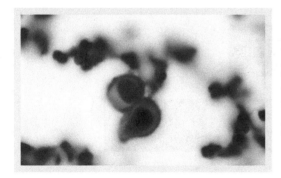

Blastomycosis

• Differentiate via culture or histopathological analysis of the organism structure.
• Broad-based budding yeasts are smaller in size.

Epidemiology

• Exposures: gardening, veterinary care, woodworking, and puncture wounds in occupational settings.
• Extracutaneous cases are rare, associated with immunosuppressed states.

Pathophysiology

• *S. schenckii* enters the skin via puncture wounds from vegetal matter (rose thorns, hay, sphagnum moss) or an infected cat, and causes a cutaneous infection at the site of inoculation.
• Lymphocutaneous disease results from lymphatic spread of the primary infection.

Clinical Features

• Subcutaneous nodules at the site of inoculation, with ulceration and central abscess formation.
• Satellite lesions develop along the path of lymphatic drainage in lymphocutaneous disease.

Special Studies

• Periodic acid–Schiff stain for organism identification (low sensitivity because of paucity of organisms).
• If no fungus is identified, sporotrichin skin test can be used to rule out infection.

Clinical Variants

• None

Good Things To Know

• Eosinophilic radiations surrounding asteroid bodies (Splendore–Hoeppli phenomenon) can be seen.

BULLOUS AND VESICULAR DERMATITIS

- **INTRAEPIDERMAL**

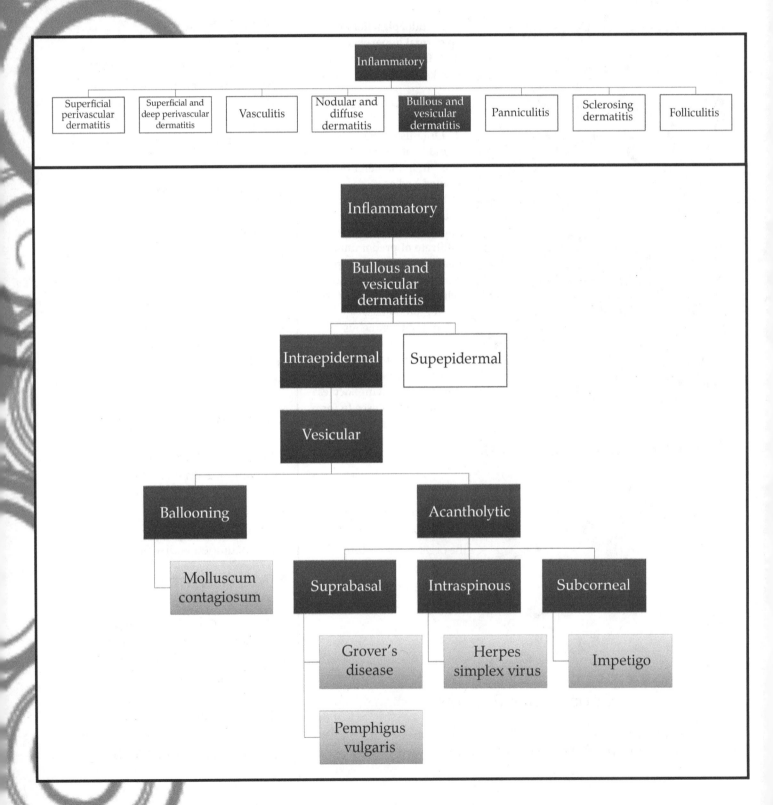

MOLLUSCUM CONTAGIOSUM

Molluscum contagiosum is a common self-limited viral infection caused by the molluscipox virus. Clinically, it presents as benign cutaneous umbilicated papules. It is histologically characterized by an acanthotic epidermis with cells containing intracytoplasmic inclusion bodies and a central keratinized crater.

HISTOLOGICAL FEATURES

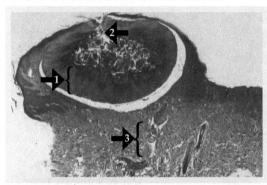

1. Epidermal acanthosis
2. Crater-shaped epithelial depression with central keratinization
3. Minimal inflammatory changes in dermis

1. Displaced nuclei
2. Large eosinophilic intracytoplasmic virion-containing inclusion bodies (molluscum bodies/Henderson–Patterson bodies) in the stratum malpighii and granulosum

HISTOLOGICAL DIFFERENTIAL

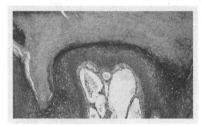

MILKER'S NODULE

• Caused by a parapoxvirus
• Acanthotic epidermis
• Marked parakeratosis
• Also has eosinophilic intracytoplasmic inclusions
• Edematous dermis with a mononuclear cell infiltrate

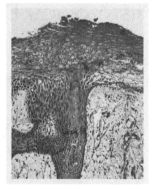

ORF

• Inter- and intracellular edema
• Ballooning degeneration
• Dense polymorphous inflammatory infiltrate
• Correlate clinically

GOOD THINGS TO KNOW
• Approximately 10% of patients develop eczematous dermatitis in areas surrounding eruptions; this subsides when the infection stops.
• HIV-infected patients can develop hundred of large lesions with little potential of self-involution.

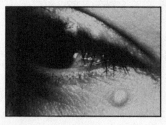

EPIDEMIOLOGY

• Common in children (age 2–5), sexually active adults, and immuno-compromised patients (e.g., HIV-infected persons).
• Most cases self-resolve within 6–9 months, but can last up to 4 years.

PATHOPHYSIOLOGY

• Belongs to the pox virus family, and has four subtypes (I–IV).
• Transmission via skin-to-skin contact and spreads with autoinoculation.
• The virus infects basal keratinocytes and causes epidermal proliferation, which results in epidermal hyperplasia and hypertrophy.

CLINICAL FEATURES

• Multiple smooth, pearly, flesh-colored papular tumors with a central white umbilication
• Size: 2–6 mm; papules enlarge as the infection progresses
• Usually asymptomatic, may be pruritic
• Commonly seen on the head, neck and trunk but may also occur on the extremities and genital area

SPECIAL STUDIES

• In situ hybridization detects the virus directly in tissue specimens.
• Geimsa stain reveals block-shaped "molluscum bodies."

CLINICAL VARIANTS

• None

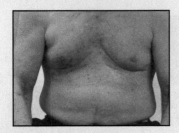

EPIDEMIOLOGY

• Mean age of 50, preferentially seen in Caucasians
• Affects men 3 times more than women
• Occurs more frequently in patients with atopic, asteatotic, and contact dermatitis

PATHOPHYSIOLOGY

• Exact etiology unknown, but proposed to be related to the obstruction of sweat ducts
• Viral, bacterial, and other pathogenic mechanisms also proposed
• Precipitating factors: strenuous exercise, sweating, excessive sun or heat exposure, and persistent fever

CLINICAL FEATURES

• Crops of discrete, skin-colored or erythematous papules or papulovesicles.
• Located on the mid-chest, central back, and proximal extremities.
• Lesions may be slightly scaly, smooth, warty, or eroded.
• Abrupt onset generally accompanied by pruritus.
• May be acute or chronic relapsing, average disease lasts 1 year.
• Typically worse in the winter months.

SPECIAL STUDIES

• Electron microscopy shows keratin filament clumping and loss of desmosomes.
• Direct immunofluorescence studies are negative.

CLINICAL VARIANTS

• None

GROVER'S DISEASE

Grover's disease, also known as transient acantholytic dermatosis, is an idiopathic, benign, self-limiting pruritic disease that commonly affects the trunk of middle-aged men. Histologically it is characterized by acantholysis, dyskeratosis, and spongiosis.

HISTOLOGICAL FEATURES

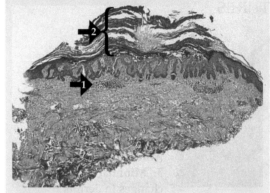

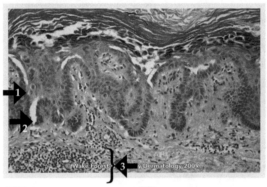

1. Lymphocytic infiltrate in superficial dermis
2. Focal hyperparakeratosis

1. Dyskeratotic keratinocyte
2. Acantholysis
3. Lymphohistiocytic infiltrate with occasional eosinophils in superficial dermis
4. Histologic patterns:
   - Darier's disease type: most common, suprabasal cleft and dyskeratosis
   - Pemphigus foliaceous type: cleft present in superficial epidermis
   - Hailey–Hailey type: cleft present throughout the stratum spinosum
   - Spongiotic type: acantholysis within vesicles

HISTOLOGICAL DIFFERENTIAL

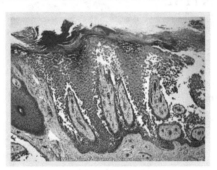

HAILEY–HAILEY

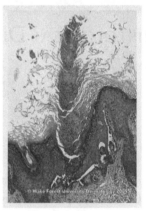

DARIER'S DISEASE

• Minimal dyskeratotic keratinocytes
• More extensive epidermal acantholysis
• Hyperplastic epidermis
• Correlate clinically

• Dyskeratotic keratinocytes
• Focal suprabasal acantholysis
• Corps ronds and corps gains
• Greater tendency to affect the hair follicles and fewer eosinophils
• Correlate clinically

GOOD THINGS TO KNOW

• The presence of spongiosis and acantholysis in the same specimen should raise the suspicion of Grover's disease.

Pemphigus Vulgaris

Pemphigus vulgaris (PV) is an autoimmune bullous disease clinically characterized by flaccid, unstable vesicles and bullae on the skin and mucous membranes. The disease is mediated by autoantibodies against desmoglein 1 and 3.

Histological Features

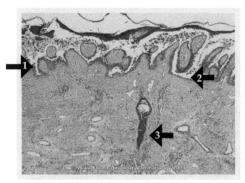

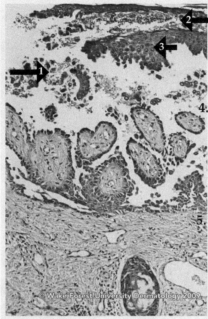

1. **Suprabasilar acantholysis**
2. **"Tombstoning" of basilar layer**
3. **Involvement of follicular structures**

1. **Acantholytic cells**
2. **Eosinophils**
3. **Spongiosis**

Other features:
Mixed papillary infiltrate with eosinophils

Histological Differential

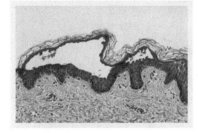

PEMPHIGUS FOLIACEOUS

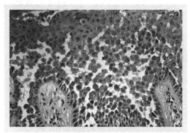

HAILEY–HAILEY DISEASE

- Autoantibodies to desmoglein 1 only
- Superficial (subcorneal/granular) epidermal cleavage
- Correlate clinically, rarely affects mucosal membranes

- Full-thickness acantholysis.
- Epidermal hyperplasia.
- Acantholysis does not affect appendageal structures (follicles).
- Negative immunofluorescence.

Good Things To Know

• Biopsies obtained from the blistered region can give false negative results; obtain sample from intact, peri-lesional skin.

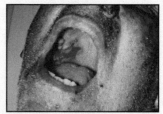

Epidemiology
• Age of onset: between 40–60 years old
• Equal male-to-female ratio
• Higher incidence in Jewish and Mediterranean populations

Pathophysiology
• IgG antibodies against desmoglein 1 and 3.
   - Desmoglein 1 is primarily expressed in the upper layers of the epidermis.
   - Desmoglein 3 is found on the spinous layer and mucous membrane.
• These antibodies interfere with calcium-dependent adhesion function and therefore induce acantholysis.

Clinical Features
• Large flaccid cutaneous bullae distributed over the face, scalp, anterior chest, intertriginous regions and pressure points.
• Lesions exhibit a positive Nikolsky sign (tangential pressure to the skin causes the blister to superficially extend).
• Mucosal lesions, particularly in the oral cavity, may be the first manifestation of disease.

Special Studies
• Direct immunofluorescence (DIF) reveals IgG1 and IgG4 deposits in the intercellular space between keratinocytes.
• Indirect immunofluorescence may reveal IgG directed against epidermal antigens.

Clinical Variants
• Pemphigus vulgaris: localized and generalized
• Pemphigus vegetans: localized
• Drug-induced

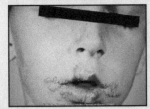

EPIDEMIOLOGY

• 8 subtypes of Human herpes virus have been defined.
  o Most are seropositive for HSV-1.
  o HSV-2 is acquired through sexual contact.
• Genital herpes is the most prevalent STD worldwide.

PATHOPHYSIOLOGY

• Transmission via contact with an infected person actively shedding the virus.
• Primarily infects nerve endings, then via retrograde transport it migrates and remains latent in the sensory/autonomic ganglia. Reactivation occurs at a later time during periods of immune compromise (common cold, menstruation, etc.).

CLINICAL FEATURES

• Typically presents as cutaneous or mucosal grouped vesicles on an erythematous base
- Prodrome of tingling/burning may precede recurrent lesions

SPECIAL STUDIES

• Tzanck smear of lesion site, but cannot distinguish between HSV-1, HSV-2, and *Varicella zoster* virus
• Serology: antibodies to glycoprotein 1 and 2 detect and differentiate between HSV-1 and HSV-2 infections
• Polymerase Chain Reaction (PCR) to detect HSV DNA in culture, smear or biopsy

CLINICAL VARIANTS

• 1° herpetic gingivostomatitis
• Herpetic labialis HSV-1
• Herpetic cervicitis
• Herpetic whitlow
• Herpes keratoconjunctivitis
• Herpes genitalia

HERPES SIMPLEX VIRUS (HSV) INFECTION

Herpes simplex virus belongs to the family Herpesviridae and has linear double-stranded DNA. Clinically, it is identified as grouped vesicles on the skin or mucous membrane, and histologically with intraepidermal vesicles, inclusion bodies, and giant keratinocytes.

HISTOLOGICAL FEATURES

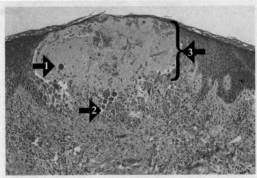

1. Multinucleated giant cell
2. Ballooning and reticular epidermal degeneration
3. Intraepidermal vesicle formation and acantholysis

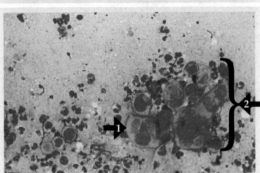

1. Multiple molded nuclei with pale chromatin
2. Multiple acantholytic balloon cells
Other features:
• Intranuclear eosinophilic inclusion bodies with clear halo (Cowdry A bodies)
• Dense lymphocytic dermal infiltrate

HISTOLOGICAL DIFFERENTIAL

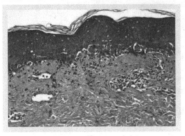

ERYTHEMA MULTIFORME

• Dyskeratotic keratinocytes
• Interface dermatitis
• Subepidermal bulla formation
• Perivascular mononuclear infiltrate

HERPES ZOSTER

• Similar epidermal changes: acantholysis, intraepidermal vesiculation, chromatic margination
• Mutinucleated giant cells

GOOD THINGS TO KNOW

• Pilosebaceous involvement is a predominant feature of herpetic folliculitis.
• HSV is the most common identifiable etiological agent in recurrent erythema multiforme.

IMPETIGO

Impetigo is a very common superficial skin infection that occurs frequently in children. Two bacterial etiologic agents are *Streptococcus* spp. and *Staphylococcus aureus*.

HISTOLOGICAL FEATURES

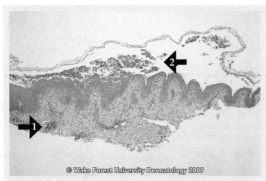

1. Mixed perivascular inflammatory infiltrate
2. Subcorneal pustules containing neutrophils and occasional acantholytic keratinocytes

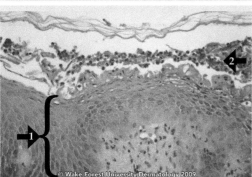

1. Spongiosis
2. Neutrophils and acantholytic keratinocytes

Other features:
• Gram positive cocci may be identified.
• Fluid filled acantholytic blister in "bullous impetigo."

HISTOLOGICAL DIFFERENTIAL

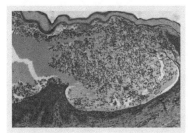

SUBCORNEAL PUSTULAR DERMATOSIS

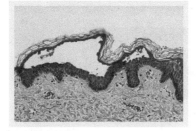

PEMPHIGUS FOLIACEUS

• Subcorneal pustules with numerous neutrophils.
• Dermal infiltrate contains few eosinophils and mononuclear cells.
• No Gram positive cocci present.
• Correlate clinically.

• Dyskeratotic granulocytes
 - Superficial subcorneal/granular epidermal cleavage.
 - DIF shows intercellular IgG deposition.

GOOD THINGS TO KNOW

• Staphylococcal scalded-skin syndrome, which is also caused by *S. aureus*, has identical histological findings to lesions of bullous impetigo.
• The infection in impetigo is limited to the epidermis; ecthyma occurs when it extends into the dermis.

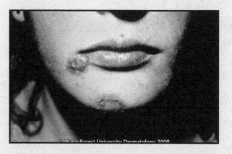

EPIDEMIOLOGY

• Most common in pre-school aged children, usually before age 2.
• Common in warm humid climates.
• 70% of cases are nonbullous.
• Contributing factors: poor hygiene, crowded living conditions, neglected skin wounds.

PATHOPHYSIOLOGY

• For primary impetigo, breaks in the skin are the main portal entry of infection.
• In secondary impetigo, a pre-existing dermatoses creates a nidus for infection.
• *S. aureus* is the most common causative agent, also group A streptococcus.

CLINICAL FEATURES

• Early lesions are vesicular in nature. The papules transform into pustules or vesicles and quickly rupture at sites of cutaneous disruption.
• Form honey-colored crusts over the site of infection.

SPECIAL STUDIES

• Gram stain: Gram positive cocci arranged in chains or clusters
• Culture of a weeping vesicle or crusted lesion

CLINICAL VARIANTS

• Bullous impetigo
• Nonbullous impetigo

BULLOUS AND VESICULAR DERMATITIS

- ## SUBEPIDERMAL

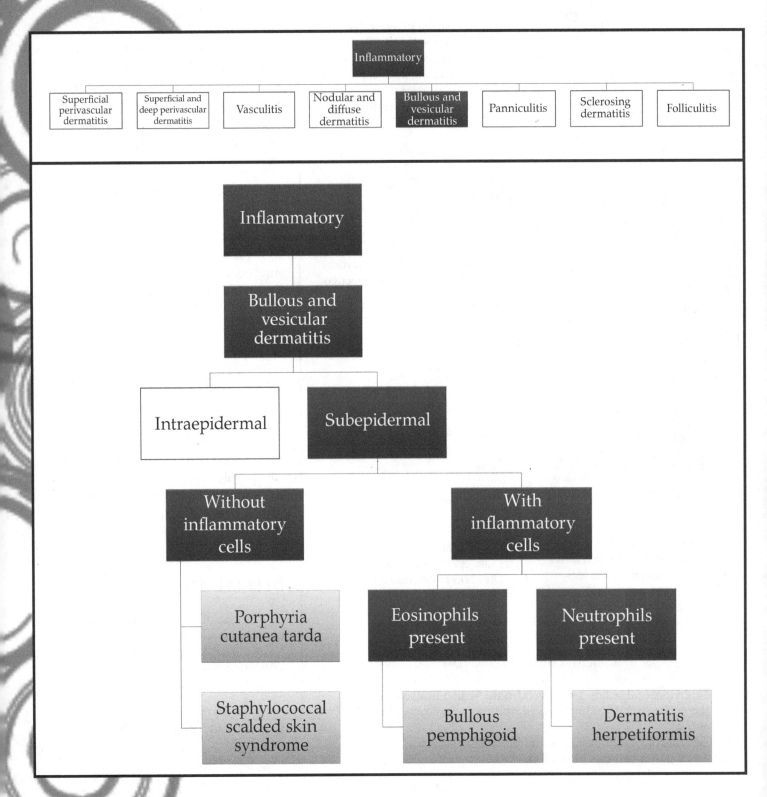

PORPHYRIA CUTANEA TARDA

Porphyria cutanea tarda (PCT) is the most common of the seven porhyrias. It is caused by an inherited or sporadic deficiency of the enzyme uroporphyrinogen decarboxylase (UROD). It is clinically characterized by blistering and fragility of sun-exposed skin.

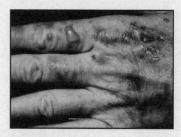

HISTOLOGICAL FEATURES

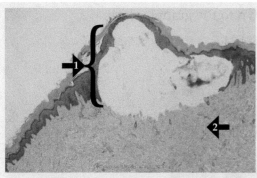

1. **Subepidermal blister**
2. **Minimal dermal inflammatory infiltrate**

1. Preserved "festooning" dermal papillae that protrude upward into the blister cavity
2. Blood vessels with thickened walls

Other features:
• Dermis shows elastosis and sclerosis of dermal collagen.
• Linear, eosinophilic, periodic acid Schiff positive globules ("caterpillar bodies") composed of basement membrane material and degenerating keratinocytes seen in the blister roof.

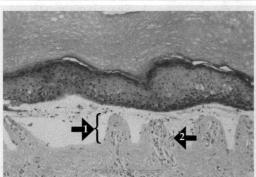

HISTOLOGICAL DIFFERENTIAL

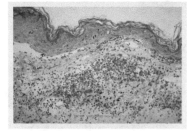

BULLOUS PEMPHIGOID

EPIDERMOLYSIS BULLOSA

• Subepidermal bullae
• Collection of eosinophils within the blister cavity
• Dense superficial dermal inflammatory infiltrate
• DIF reveals linear IgG and C3 deposits along the DEJ

• Noninflammatory subepidermal bullae
• No dermal vascular wall thickening
• Correlate clinically

GOOD THINGS TO KNOW

• PCT is not an autoimmune disorder; the IgG deposits seen on immunofluorescence studies are believed to be immunoproteins that leaked out of the damaged vasculature.

EPIDEMIOLOGY

• More common in 30 to 50 year olds
• Equal incidence in males and females

PATHOPHYSIOLOGY

• The deficient enzyme, UROD, is the 5th enzyme in the heme biosynthetic pathway.
• Leads to accumulation of uroporphyrin and porphyrins.
• It is hypothesized that sun exposure causes the activated porphyrins in the skin to release cytokines and cause vascular damage.
• The subepidermal blisters form secondary to immunoglobulin deposition in the vascular walls.

CLINICAL FEATURES

• Increased fragility of sun-exposed skin, especially the back of hands and forearms
• Painful bullae and vesicles
• Resolve with atrophic scars, milia and mottled hyper- and hypopigmention
• Hypertrichosis of upper face and forehead

SPECIAL STUDIES

• Direct immunofluorescence studies reveal linear IgG and C3 deposits around the superficial vascular vessels.
• Elevated urine porphyrins.
• Wood lamp exam of urine reveals a orange-red fluorescence.

CLINICAL VARIANTS

• Type I (sporadic) – acquired and restricted to liver
• Type II (familial) – hereditary and present in all the tissues
• Type III (rare) - hereditary and localized to the liver

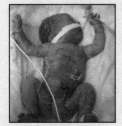

EPIDEMIOLOGY

• Equal sex distribution
• Common in newborns and children <5 years
• Can occur in adults with severe underlying disease: systemic immuno-suppresion, renal failure, etc.

PATHOPHYSIOLOGY

• From the site of infection, *S. aureus* releases toxins that are systemically absorbed.
• Exotoxin A and B are superantigens that activate the immune response by activating major histocompatibility complex class II molecules on the antigen presenting cells.
• This results in a massive flux of cytokines larger than what would be seen with a typical antigen-specific activation.

CLINICAL FEATURES

• Patients are acutely ill presenting with a high fever.
• Cutaneous lesions start as a sunburn-like rash with diffuse erythema, and progress to flaccid blisters that easily rupture.
• Large areas of the superficial epidermis separate and slough off.

SPECIAL STUDIES

• A new rapid serum test to detect the toxin
• Frozen section of sloughed off skin to determine the site of separation cleavage

CLINICAL VARIANTS

• None

STAPHYLOCOCCAL SCALDED-SKIN SYNDROME (SSSS)

SSSS is an acute systemic illness that results from the release of exfoliative exotoxins by certain strains of *Staphylococcus aureus*. Clinically, widespread erythema and formation and rupture of bullae are seen. Histologically, it is characterized by subcorneal bullae that may extend down to the granular layer.

HISTOLOGICAL FEATURES

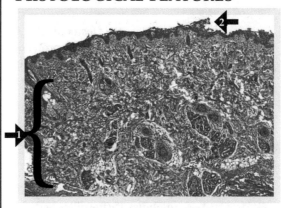

1. Spare lymphocytic dermal infiltrate
2. Sloughing of the epidermis

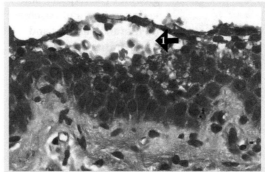

1. Subcorneal blister containing acantholytic keratinocytes

Other features:
• No bacteria detectable in lesions

HISTOLOGICAL DIFFERENTIAL

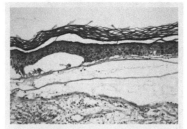

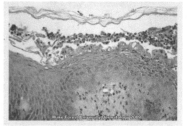

TOXIC EPIDERMAL NECROLYSIS
• Involves more extensive epidermal necrosis
• Minimal inflammatory infiltrate with occasional eosinophils

BULLOUS IMPETIGO
• Subcorneal pustules
• Fluid-filled acantholytic blister
• Gram positive cocci may be identified
• Epidermal spongiosis

GOOD THINGS TO KNOW

• The target of the exotoxins is desmoglein 1, which is also the target site of the toxin in bullous impetigo and the IgG antibody in pemphigus foliaceus.

BULLOUS PEMPHIGOID (BP)

Bullous pemphigoid is an autoimmune disease characterized by tense cutaneous bullae on an erythematous base. It is histologically characterized by subepidermal blisters that are mediated by IgG antibodies against hemidesmosomal proteins in the epidermis.

HISTOLOGICAL FEATURES

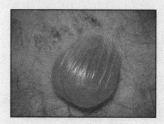

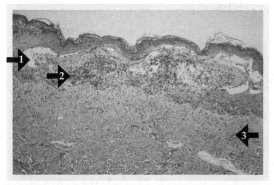

1. **Subepidermal blister**
2. **Eosinophils and lymphocytes in blister cavity**
3. **Perivascular lymphocytic infiltrate**

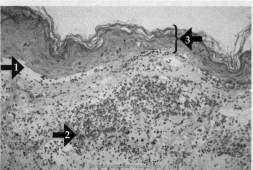

1. **Subepidermal blister**
2. **Eosinophilic infiltrate**
3. **Normal overlying epithelium**

HISTOLOGICAL DIFFERENTIAL

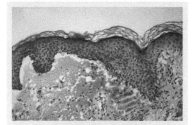

EPIDERMOLYSIS BULLOSA ACQUISITA (EBA)

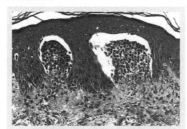

DERMATITIS HERPETIFORMIS

- Subepidermal bullae.
- Less eosinophilic infiltrate in subepidermis.
- In salt-split skin, immunofluorescence reveals IgG deposits in the blister base.

- Subepidermal blisters
- Predominance of neutrophils in the dermal papillae
- Granular IgA deposits in superficial papillary dermis on DIF

GOOD THINGS TO KNOW

- Other dermatoses that exhibit eosinophilic spongiosis include incontinentia pigmenti, pemphigus, contact dermatitis, and arthropod bite.
- Indirect immunofluorescence reveals circulating autoantibodies in the serum of 60–80% of patients; however, the titer does not correlate to disease severity.

EPIDEMIOLOGY

- Occurs primarily in the elderly
- Equal sex distribution
- No racial predilection

PATHOPHYSIOLOGY

- Immunoglobulins target hemidesmosomal proteins, BP230 and BP180, located at the epidermal-dermal junction.
- Activates the complement cascade, the release of cytokines attracts an inflammatory infiltrate.
- Neutrophils and eosinophils release lysosomal proteolytic enzymes that cause subepidermal blister formation.

CLINICAL FEATURES

- Tense cutaneous blisters on an erythematous base or normal skin
- Blisters are dense and intact, exhibit a negative Nikolsky's sign
- Diffuse distribution, but have a predilection for the extremities
- Asymptomatic to severe pruritis

SPECIAL STUDIES

- Direct immunofluorescence (DIF) of peri-lesional skin reveals linear C3 and immunoglobin deposit along the epidermal–dermal junction.
- Indirect immunofluorescence (IDIF) of salt-split skin reveals IgG deposits on the roof of blisters.

CLINICAL VARIANTS

- None

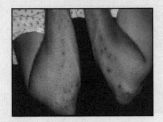

EPIDEMIOLOGY

• The prevalence of DH in various Caucasian populations varies between 10 and 39/100,000 persons, highest in Scandinavia.
• Can present at any age, most common in 20–30s.
• Male:female ratio is 2:1.

PATHOPHYSIOLOGY

• An autoimmune-mediated disease caused by IgA antibodies against tissue transglutaminase.
• This results in activation of the immune cascade causing neutrophil recruitment and complement activation.

CLINICAL FEATURES

• Intensely pruritic, chronic papulovesicular eruption.
• Lesions are grouped with small crusted erosions secondary to excoriation.
• Symmetrical distribution over extensor surfaces of extremities.
• The typical distribution of lesions is over the buttocks, shoulders, and elbows.

SPECIAL STUDIES

• DIF studies show granular deposits of IgA along the dermal papillae.
• Circulating anti-endomysium antibodies and antibodies to tissue transglutaminase are present in 90% of cases.

CLINICAL VARIANTS

• None

DERMATITIS HERPETIFORMIS

Dermatitis herpetiformis (DH) is an uncommon autoimmune disease that manifests as an intensely puritic skin eruption. It is associated with gluten-sensitive enteropathy, known as celiac disease.

HISTOLOGICAL FEATURES

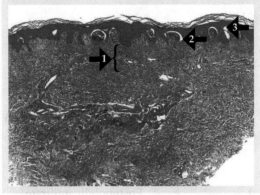

1. Lymphocytic infiltrate surrounding superficial dermal vasculature
2. Subepidermal bullae
3. Microabcess in tips of dermal papillae

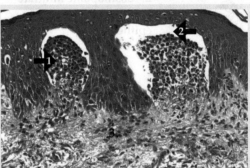

1. Discrete collection of neutrophils localized in the dermal papillae tips
2. Subepidermal bullae
Other features:
• Excoriated epidermis

HISTOLOGICAL DIFFERENTIAL

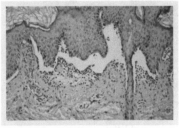

LINEAR IGA BULLOUS DERMATOSIS
• Subepidermal bullae
• Neutrophilic infiltrate distributed along the dermal–epidermal junction
• DIF: IgA antibodies in a linear/granular pattern against the basement membrane

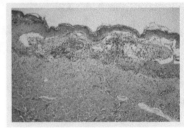

BULLOUS PEMPHIGOID
• Subepidermal bullae.
• Collection of eosinophils within the blister cavity.
• Dense superficial dermal inflammatory infiltrate.
• DIF reveals linear IgG and C3 deposits along the DEJ.

GOOD THINGS TO KNOW
• The rash responds rapidly to dapsone therapy. Strict adherence to a gluten-free diet is also effective.
• Active blisters are rarely seen because of the associated itching and excoriation.
• Associated with HLA antigens -B8, -DR3, and -DQ2.

PANNICULITIS

- **SEPTAL**
- **LOBULAR**

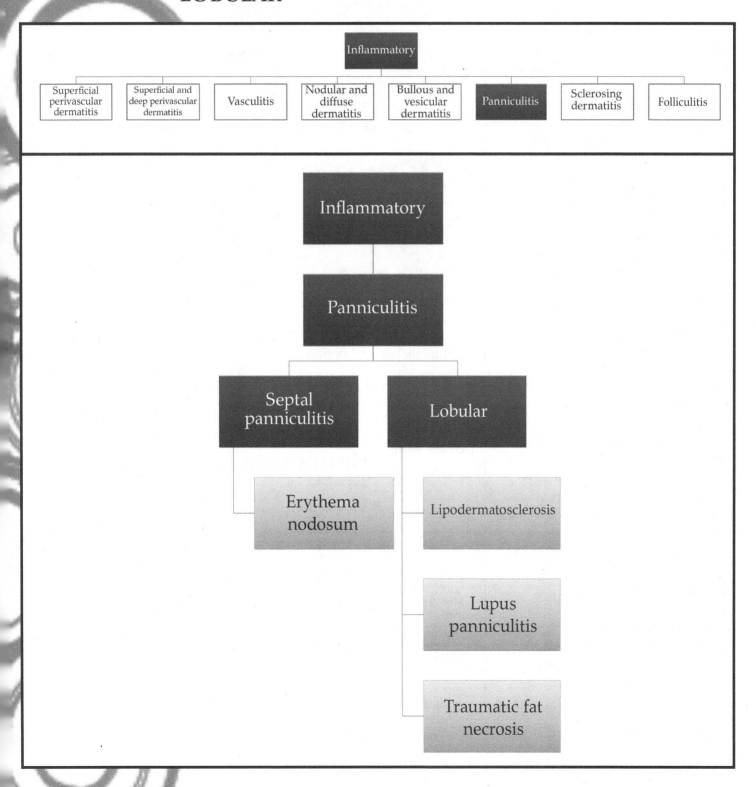

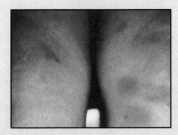

EPIDEMIOLOGY

• Common causes include: infections (*Yersinia*), drugs (oral contraceptives), inflammatory diseases (ulcerative colitis), and granulomatous disorders (Sarcoidosis).
• Peak age is between 20–30 years old.
• Equal incidence prior to puberty, with a female predominance after puberty.

PATHOPHYSIOLOGY

• Erythema nodosum is considered to be a delayed hypersensitivity response to a variety of eliciting agents.

CLINICAL FEATURES

• Acute onset of symmetrical, well-localized, tender, erythematous, warm nodules.
• Usually located on the extensor surface of lower extremities, ankles, and knees.
• Late stages may appear as a deep bruise ("erythema contusiformis").
• May be accompanied with low-grade fever, fatigue, malaise, arthralgias especially of the ankles and knees.

SPECIAL STUDIES

• Elevated laboratory studies: erythrocyte sedimentation rate, C-reactive protein, leukocytosis

CLINICAL VARIANTS

• None

ERYTHEMA NODOSUM

Erythema nodosum is a septal panniculitis involving the subcutaneous fat and manifests as an acute eruption of tender nodules that is triggered by or associated with various conditions.

HISTOLOGICAL FEATURES

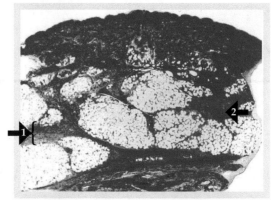

1. **Thickened septa**
2. **Peripheral inflammatory infiltrate surrounding fat lobules**

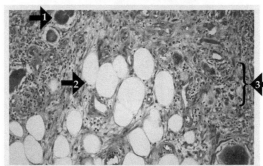

1. **Multinucleated giant cells**
2. **Adipose cells**
3. **Inflammatory cell infiltrate**

• Early lesions:
  - Lymphocytic (initially neutrophilic) dermal perivascular infiltrate
  - Septal polymorphous infiltration in fat lobules that can extend to the paraseptal regions between individual adipocytes in a lace-like manner

• Chronic lesions:
  - Granulomatous panniculitis
  - Miescher's radial granulomas, nodular aggregrations of histiocytes situated radially around a central cleft
  - Thickened and fibrosed fat septa

HISTOLOGICAL DIFFERENTIAL

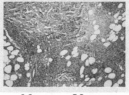

NODULAR VASCULITIS
• Lobular panniculitis.
• Mixed perivascular infiltrate in deep dermis.
• Fat necrosis may be present.
• Vasculitis of deep dermal and septal arteries.

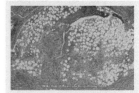

TRAUMATIC PANNICULITIS
• Lobular infiltrate of foamy histiocytes and multinucleated giant cells
• Encapsulated fat necrosis surrounded by fibrosis (micropseudocysts)
• Erythrocyte extravasation

GOOD THINGS TO KNOW
• Biopsy should be obtained from the central portion of the lesion and must include subcutaneous fat.
• Vasculitis is not a major feature, but thrombophlebitis and minimal vascular damage can be seen.

LIPODERMATOSCLEROSIS

Lipodermatosclerosis, also known as sclerosing panniculitis and hypodermatitis sclerodermaformis is a form of pannicultis (septal and lobular) that typically occurs on the lower extremities on women with a history of venous insufficiency and stasis.

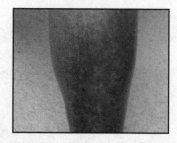

HISTOLOGICAL FEATURES

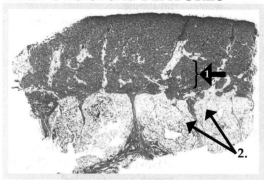

1. **Hyalinized fibrous tissue**
2. **Obliteration of fat lobules**

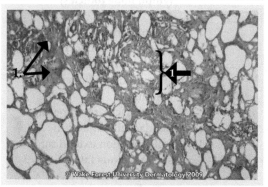

1. **Obliteration of fat lobules by hyalinized fibrous tissue**
2. **Lipomembranous fat necrosis: fat lobules with ghost cells (pale cells with absent nuclei)**
Other features:
• **Perivascular lymphocytic infiltrate**
• **Chronic stage: extensive fibrosis and sclerosis with minimal inflammation**

HISTOLOGICAL DIFFERENTIAL

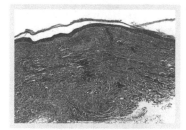

LUPUS PANNICULITIS

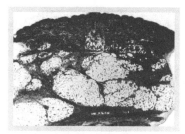

ERYTHEMA NODOSUM

• Epidermal atrophy
• Hyaline necrosis of fat lobules
• Hyalinization of surrounding connective tissue
• Paraseptal lymphoid follicles

• Septal polymorphous (initially neutrophilic) infiltrate in fat lobules
• Granulomatous panniculitis
• Thickened and fibrosed septa
• Correlate clinically

GOOD THINGS TO KNOW

• Biopsy should be avoided as skin wounds heal poorly.

EPIDEMIOLOGY

• Most commonly diagnosed in middle-aged women.
• Two-thirds of patients are obese.
• Usually seen in patients with a history of
  - Venous insufficiency
  - Stasis and varicosities
  - Thromboses

PATHOPHYSIOLOGY

• Venous incompetency, venous hypertension, and obesity play a role in etiology.
• Stasis causes decreased perfusion of lobular capillaries, resulting in ischemia and centrolobular fat necrosis.
• Venous hypertension causes diffusion of substances, like fibrin, out of capillaries, which predisposes tissue to ulceration.

CLINICAL FEATURES

• Lesions progress, and have a brown-red pigmentation (hemosiderin deposition), more severe induration with lichenification, edema, atrophie blanche, varicose veins, and ulcerations.
• Most commonly affects the distal third lower extremities, "champagne bottle or bowling pin" sign.

SPECIAL STUDIES

• None

CLINICAL VARIANTS

• None

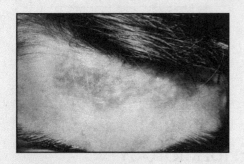

EPIDEMIOLOGY

• Seen primarily in adults
• More common in females (F:M, 2:1)
• 10–50% of patients with lupus panniculitis have or eventually develop systemic lupus erythematosus

PATHOPHYSIOLOGY

• Variant of lupus erythematosus, involving the subcutaneous fat.
• 2–5% of patients with SLE have concomitant lesion of lupus panniculitis.

CLINICAL FEATURES

• Deep, erythematous plaques and nodules often with ulcers.
• Can involve the face, proximal extremities, shoulders, trunk, breasts, and buttocks.
• Lesions are typically painful and frequently heal with atrophy and scarring.
• May also have lesions of discoid lupus erythematosus.

SPECIAL STUDIES

• Serological studies are generally negative, but antinuclear antibody titers may occasionally be positive.

CLINICAL VARIANTS

• None

LUPUS PANNICULITIS

Lupus panniculitis, also known as lupus profundus, is a variant of lupus erythematosus involving the subcutaneous fat. It is clinically characterized by diffuse indurated subcutaneous nodules or plaques. Histologically, it involves panniculitis of the septal and lobular regions.

HISTOLOGICAL FEATURES

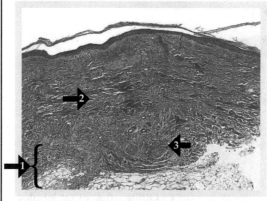

1. Hyalinizing necrosis of fat lobule
2. Dermal mucinous edema
3. Dense lymphocytic infiltrate

~~~~~~~~~~~~~~~~~~~~~~~~~~~~~~~~~~~~

1. Hyalinization of connective tissue, blood vessels, and fat lobules
2. Nodular aggregates of lymphocytes surrounded by plasma cells (may resemble lymph node follicles)

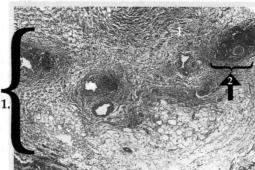

Other features:
• Mixed lymphocytic septal-lobular panniculitis surrounding adipocytes (rimming)
• Perivascular and periappendageal lymphocytic inflammation extending into subcutaneous fat

HISTOLOGICAL DIFFERENTIAL

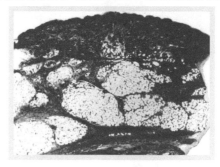

ERYTHEMA NODOSUM
• Septal polymorphous panniculitis
• Thickened and fibrosed septa
• Correlate clinically

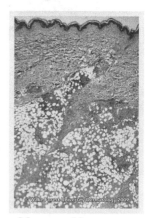

NODULAR VASCULITIS
• Polymorphous lobular panniculitis.
• Mixed perivascular infiltrate in deep dermis.
• Fat necrosis may be present.

GOOD THINGS TO KNOW
• Rarity of involvement of the lower extremities distinguishes this condition from other forms of panniculitis, particularly erythema nodosum.
• Lupus panniculitis can occur as a primary separate entity or in association with systemic lupus erythematosus or discoid lupus erythematosus.

Traumatic Fat Necrosis

Trauma is a common cause of subcutaneous fat necrosis, resulting either from surgery or an external assault.

Histological Features

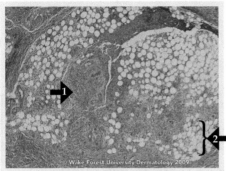

1. Mixed inflammatory infiltrate
2. Nonspecific fat necrosis

1. Normal epidermis
2. Lobular panniculitis

Other features:
• Early lesions show nonspecific lobular and septal fat necrosis.
• Cystic spaces with adjacent general inflammatory infiltrate including macrophages, lymphocytes, and neutrophils in adipose tissue.
• Perivascular lymphocytic infiltrates at the dermal–subcutaneous interface
• Multinucleated giant cells like a

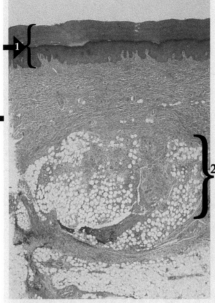

foreign body granuloma.
• Hemosiderin-laden macrophages present in traumatic lesions.
• Can also see foam cell collections and calcium deposits.

Histological Differential

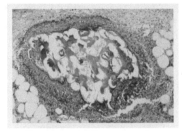

Pancreatic Panniculitis

• Necrotic adipocytes with thickened cell walls and no nuclei (ghost cells)
• Calcifications and enzymatic fat necrosis (saponification)
• Neutrophilic infiltrate, later replaced with a monocytic, granulomatous inflammation

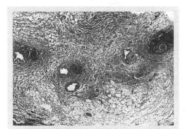

Lupus Panniculitis

• Hyaline necrosis of fat lobules
• Hyalinization of surrounding connective tissue
• Paraseptal lymphoid follicles
• Perivascular lymphoplasma-cytic infiltrate

Good Things To Know

• Trauma-related panniculitis of the breasts can produce lesions with a peau d'orange appearance secondary to skin retractions, mimicking malignancy.

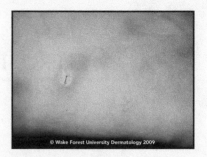

Epidemiology

• The injurious incident may be secondary to an accidental or iatrogenic event.
• Infants are at the highest risk for cold panniculitis.
• Sclerosing lipogranuloma is seen most commonly in young adults.

Pathophysiology

• Trauma causes necrosis of the subcutaneous fat.
• Lipases secreted from adipocytes release free fatty acids that combine with calcium to produce detergents.
• This sets up a foreign body. granuloma reaction to destroy the fat tissue.

Clinical Features

• Erythematous, tender, indurated plaques 2–3 days after exposure in cold panniculitis.
- In sclerosing lipogranuloma, implantation of foreign material causes lesions related to the properties of the implicated substance.
- Inciting trauma not often recalled.

Special Studies

• Polarized microscopy to identify foreign materials

Clinical Variants

• Cold panniculitis
• Sclerosing lipogranuloma
• Chemical panniculitis
• Trauma-related panniculitis

Inflammatory

| Superficial perivascular dermatitis | Superficial and deep perivascular dermatitis | Vasculitis | Nodular and diffuse dermatitis | Bullous and vesicular dermatitis | Panniculitis | Sclerosing dermatitis | Folliculitis |

Inflammatory

Sclerosing dermatitis

Morphea

Morphea

Morphea is a subtype of scleroderma that is limited to the skin and subcutaneous tissue. It is a chronic sclerosing dermatitis that clinically presents as indurated sclerotic plaques with a violaceous border.

Histological Features

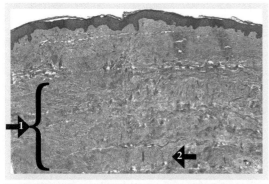

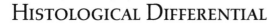

1. Sclerotic reticular dermis with hyperplastic widened collagen bundles arranged in parallel fashion
2. Minimal inflammatory infiltrate

1. Hyperplastic collagen bundles.
2. Elastic stains reveal thick elastin fibers arranged parallel to the collagen strands.
Other features:
• Normal to atrophic epidermis
• Diffuse perivascular inflammatory infiltrate containing plasma cells and occasional eosinophils
• Sclerotic involvement of adnexal structures

Histological Differential

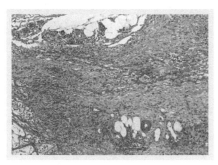

EOSINOPHILIC FASCIITIS

• Inflammation, edema, and sclerosis of the fascia
• Mixed cellular infiltrate consisting of lymphocytes, plasma cells, histiocytes, and eosinophils

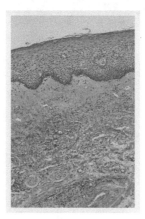

LICHEN SCLEROSUS ET ATROPHICUS

• Thinning of rete in epidermis
• Prominent papillary dermal sclerosis
• Uninvolved reticular dermis

Good Things To Know
• There is ≤ 1% chance of progression of morphea to systemic scleroderma.
• Morphea and cutaneous scleroderma demonstrate similar histological features.
  o Early lesions of morphea exhibit greater inflammatory infiltrate and more edema.

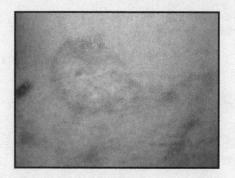

Epidemiology

• Onset between 20–50 years old
• More common in females (F:M, 3:1)
• More common in Caucasians

Pathophysiology

• The exact cause is unknown, but ought to be immunologically mediated
• Patients have an increased number of fibroblasts and an increased rate of collagen biosynthesis in the skin.
• Proposed to be related to *Borrelia burgdorferi* infection.

Clinical Features

• Solitary or multiple sclerotic, indurated plaques.
• Central hypopigmentation with a red-violaceous border (lilac ring).
• Lesions can persist for 3–5 years with eventual improvement, but often leave hyperpigmented skin patches.

Special Studies

• Serological testing to rule out *B. burgdorferi* infection

Clinical Variants

• Circumscribed
• Macular
• Linear
• Frontoparietal
• Generalized
• Pansclerotic

FOLLICULITIS

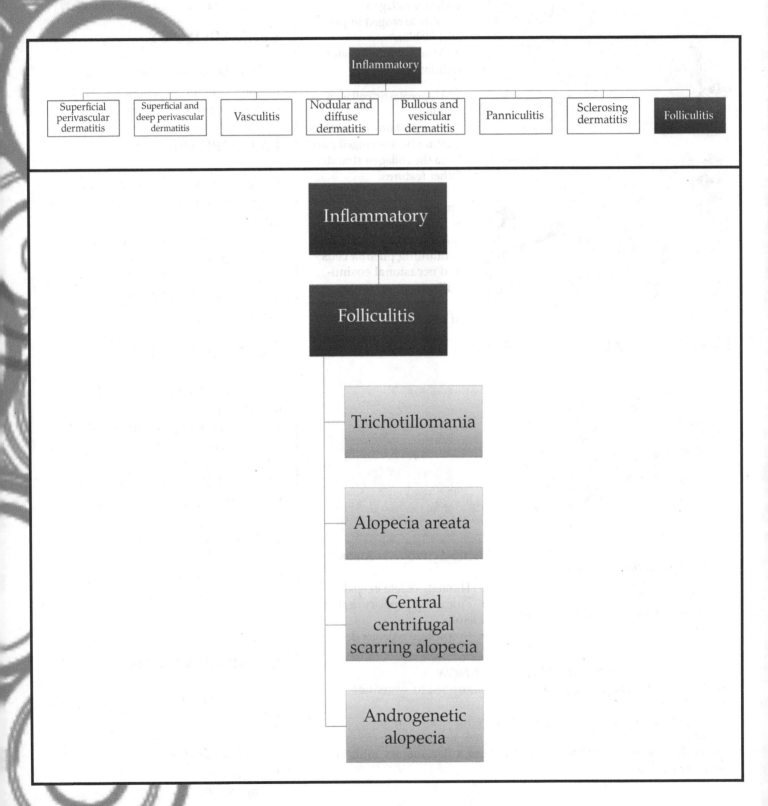

TRICHOTILLOMANIA

Trichotillomania is a self-induced, poorly demarcated alopecia due to compulsions that cause individuals to pull out their hair. In children, this is often a habit that is outgrown, whereas in adults, this may represent an underlying psychiatric illness.

HISTOLOGICAL FEATURES

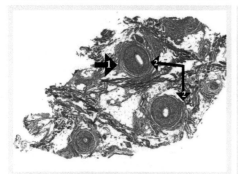

1. **Minimal inflammatory infiltrate**
2. **Empty dilated hair follicles**

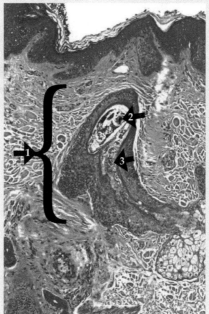

1. **Trichomalacia (soft, pigmented and distorted hair shafts)**
2. **Pigment casts**
3. **Distorted hair canal**
Other features:
• **Broken hair with perifollicular hemorrhage.**
• **Empty anagen hair follicles, with an increased number of catagen hair follicles, are seen simultaneously.**

HISTOLOGICAL DIFFERENTIAL

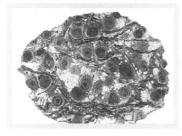

ALOPECIA AREATA

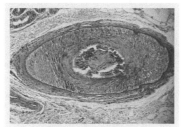

TINEA CAPITIS

• Increased terminal catagen and telogen hairs
• Decrease terminal anagen hairs
• Perifollicular mononuclear inflammatory cell infiltrate

• Fungal stains reveal spores and hyphae present in the hair and stratum corneum.
• Chronic folliculitis with intra-follicular neutrophils.
• May present as a granulomatous reaction.

GOOD THINGS TO KNOW

• Biopsy should be done on most recent patches to obtain best histologic findings.

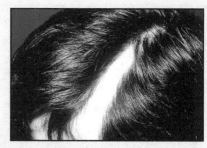

EPIDEMIOLOGY

• Incidence of 0.6–3.4% in American adults.
• Predisposing factors include a history of psychiatric illness.
• Childhood trichotillomania is often found equally amongst boys and girls.
• Adult trichotillomania is found more often in women.

PATHOPHYSIOLOGY

• Traumatic alopecia resulting secondary to compulsions involving pulling, rubbing or twisting of the hair

CLINICAL FEATURES

• Ill-circumscribed areas of incomplete to complete alopecia.
• Scalp is usually not scarred.
• Broken hairs can be seen alongside newly growing hair.
• The most common area affected is the scalp.
• Less often, eyebrows, eyelashes and pubic hair may be affected.

SPECIAL STUDIES

• PAS and silver stains to identify/rule out fungi associated with tinea capitis

CLINICAL VARIANTS

• None

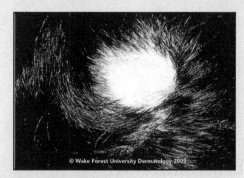

EPIDEMIOLOGY

• Primarily affects children and young adults <25 years old
• 10-20% have a familial history
• More common in females
• Associated with other autoimmune diseases

PATHOPHYSIOLOGY

• Multifactorial etiology:
  o Immune-mediated, genetics, and environmental triggers
• Possible triggers include infections, emotional stress, seasonal variations

CLINICAL FEATURES

• Patchy areas of circumscribed hair loss.
• Broken, fractured "exclamation point" hairs at the spreading margin.
• Occurs most commonly on the scalp, but can be seen localized to the eyebrows, beard, and body hair.
• Underlying skin appears normal with minimal erythema and has follicular openings.

SPECIAL STUDIES

• None

CLINICAL VARIANTS

• Alopecia areata totalis – complete loss of scalp hair
• Alopecia areata universalis – complete loss of body hair

ALOPECIA AREATA

Alopcia areata (AA) is an inflammatory reversible non-scarring alopecia. It has an unpredictable clinical course, ranging from self-limited spontaneous resolution to severe recurrent chronic disease. For some patients, it has a major impact on their quality of life.

HISTOLOGICAL FEATURES

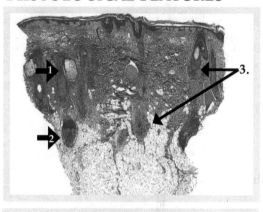

1. Miniaturized hair follicle
2. Telogen hair follicle with surrounding inflammation
3. Peribulbar lymphocytic infiltrate

1. Perifollicular lymphocytic infiltrate
2. "Swarm of bees" appearance
Other features:
• Decreased terminal hairs, increased vellus hairs
• Decreased anagen hairs
• High percentage of catagen and telogen hairs
• Degenerative changes in hair matrix
• May find pigment casts in the papillary dermis and follicular stelae

HISTOLOGICAL DIFFERENTIAL

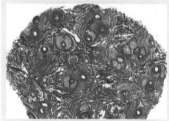

ANDROGENETIC ALOPECIA

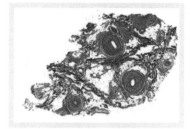

TRICHOTILLOMANIA

• Decreased catagen hairs
• Follicular miniaturization
• No pigment casts

• Increased catagen hairs and empty follicles
• Pigment casts in follicular channels
• No follicular miniaturization
• No inflammatory infiltrate

GOOD THINGS TO KNOW

• Obtaining two perspectives of scalp biopsies, including horizontal and vertical sections, helps narrow the differential and reach the correct diagnosis.

CENTRAL CENTRIFUGAL SCARRING ALOPECIA

Central centrifugal scarring alopecia (CCSA) is an idiopathic progressive scarring alopecia most commonly seen in African American women. Clinically it is characterized by vertex-centered alopecia, and perifollicular fibrosis is seen on histological analysis.

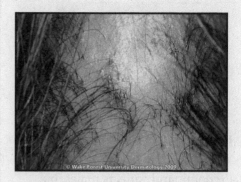

HISTOLOGICAL FEATURES

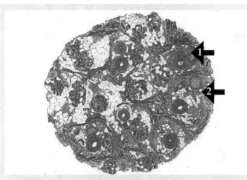

1. & 2. Fibrosis surrounding hair follicle

1. **Perifollicular lymphocytic infiltrate at the level of the infundibulum**
2. **Perifollicular fibrosis**

Other features:
• **At areas of destroyed follicle, residual fibrotic tracks may be seen.**

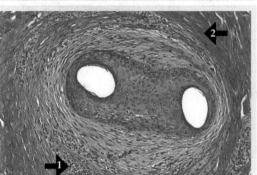

HISTOLOGICAL DIFFERENTIAL

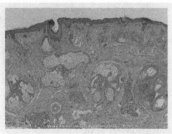

DISCOID LUPUS ERYTHEMATOSUS (DLE)

• Very similar in histological appearance.
• Mucin deposits seen within collagen strands.
• Interface dermatitis more commonly seen in DLE.

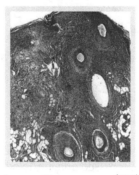

LICHEN PLANOPILARIS (LPP)

• Very similar in histological appearance.
• Interface dermatitis more commonly seen in LPP.
• Clinical correlation is usually necessary.

EPIDEMIOLOGY

• Common in African American women
• Female:male ratio about 3:1 in the African American population

PATHOPHYSIOLOGY

• Usually patients report a history of using chemical hair treatments.
• Anatomic abnormality causes premature desquamation of the inner root sheath and resulting inflammatory changes or injury.

CLINICAL FEATURES

• Scarring typically seen on the central scalp and expands centrifugally.
• Usually asymptomatic.

SPECIAL STUDIES

• None

CLINICAL VARIANTS

• None

GOOD THINGS TO KNOW

• Horizontal sections are usually required for diagnosis.

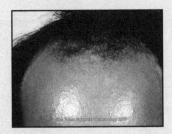

EPIDEMIOLOGY

• Onset generally in 20s or early 30s.
• Predominantly affects males, but females can be affected.

ETIOLOGY

• Exact mechanism is unknown; however, inherited factors and effects of androgens on the hair follicle are responsible.
• Autosomal dominance with variable penetrance and multifactorial inheritance has been suggested as the genetic contributing factor.

PATHOPHYSIOLOGY

• It is recognized that both genetic and androgenic factors are involved.
• In genetically predisposed individuals, dihydrotestosterone (DHT) transforms terminal hair follicles into vellus-like follicles.
• The telogen phase lengthens and the anagen phase becomes shorter.
• Over time the follicles become short and small, with sclerosis of the dermis and a reduction in the diameter of hairs present.

CLINICAL FEATURES

• Males: receding frontal hairline, particularly over the parietal and temporal areas; circular patch of hair loss over the vertex
• Females: intact frontal hairline with diffuse thinning and hair loss over the top of the scalp in a "christmas tree" pattern

SPECIAL STUDIES

• None

CLINICAL VARIANTS

• None

ANDROGENETIC ALOPECIA

Androgenetic alopecia, commonly referred to as pattern baldness, is characterized by a gradual loss of hair mainly from the vertex and frontotemporal regions of the scalp secondary to hormonal factors and a genetic predisposition.

HISTOLOGICAL FEATURES

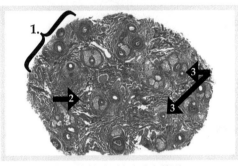

1. **Normal number of total follicles.**
2. **Variable perifollicular lymphohistiocytic inflammation may be seen.**
3. **Miniaturized hair follicles with variable diameter.**

1. **Prominent sebaceous glands**
2. **Follicular stelae**
Other features:
• **Decreased terminal hairs, increased vellus hairs and follicular stelae**
• **Decreased anagen/telogen ratio**

HISTOLOGICAL DIFFERENTIAL

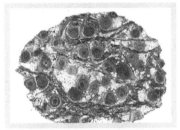

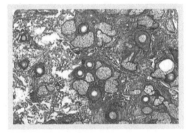

ALOPECIA AREATA

• Miniaturized hair follicles
• Decreased anagen/telogen ratio
• Peribulbar lymphocytic infiltrate surrounding follicles

TELOGEN EFFLUVIUM

• No diminution in follicular or hair shaft size.
• Normal numbers of terminal and vellus hairs and follicular stelae
• Increased number of telogen hairs during active phase

GOOD THINGS TO KNOW

• A terminal–vellus ratio of less than 4:1 indicates follicular miniaturization.
• Variation in hair shaft diameter is best assessed in horizontal sections.

APPENDIX

- DERMATOPATHOLOGY HIERARCHY INFRASTRUCTURE
- GLOSSARY OF TERMS
- BIBLIOGRAPHY

Lymphohistiocytic dermatitis

Dermatopathology hierarchy infrastructure

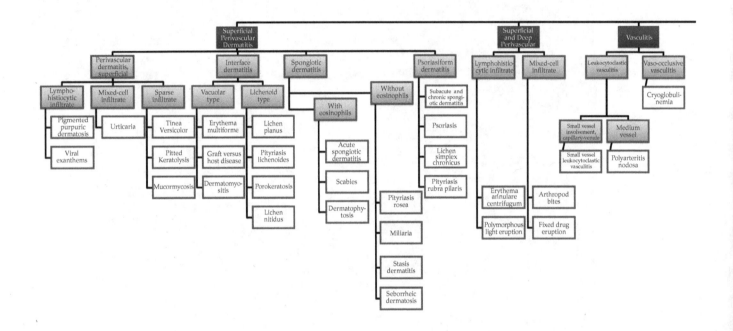

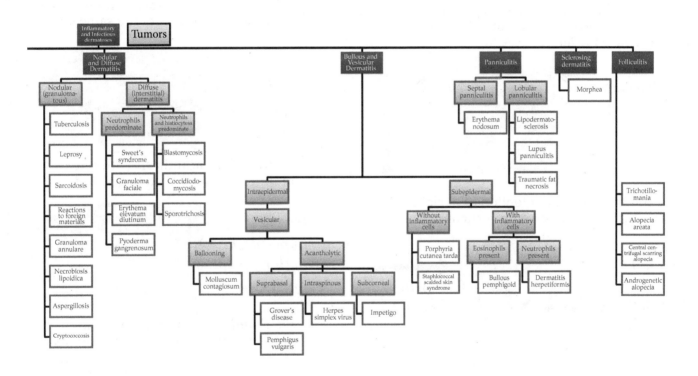

Inflammatory and Infectious dermatoses

Tumors

Nodular and Diffuse Dermatitis

- Nodular (granulomatous)
  - Tuberculosis
  - Leprosy
  - Sarcoidosis
  - Reactions to foreign materials
  - Granuloma annulare
  - Necrobiosis lipoidica
  - Aspergillosis
  - Cryptococcosis
- Diffuse (interstitial) dermatitis
  - Neutrophils predominate
    - Sweet's syndrome
    - Granuloma faciale
    - Erythema elevatum diutinum
    - Pyoderma gangrenosum
  - Neutrophils and histiocytes predominate
    - Blastomycosis
    - Coccidiodomycosis
    - Sporotrichosis

Bullous and Vesicular Dermatitis

- Intraepidermal
  - Vesicular
    - Ballooning
      - Molluscum contagiosum
    - Acantholytic
      - Suprabasal
        - Grover's disease
        - Pemphigus vulgaris
      - Intraspinous
        - Herpes simplex virus
      - Subcorneal
        - Impetigo
- Subepidermal
  - Without inflammatory cells
    - Porphyria cutanea tarda
    - Staphlococcal scalded skin syndrome
  - With inflammatory cells
    - Eosinophils present
      - Bullous pemphigoid
    - Neutrophils present
      - Dermatitis herpetiformis

Panniculitis

- Septal panniculitis
  - Erythema nodosum
- Lobular panniculitis
  - Lipodermatosclerosis
  - Lupus panniculitis
  - Traumatic fat necrosis

Sclerosing dermatitis

- Morphea

Folliculitis

- Trichotillomania
- Alopecia areata
- Central centrifugal scarring alopecia
- Androgenetic alopecia

GLOSSARY OF TERMS

EPIDERMAL

a. **Hyperkeratosis** - thickening of the stratum corneum

Hyperkeratosis

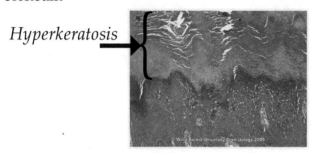

b. **Orthokeratosis** - "basket-weave" appearance of the stratum corneum without retention of keratinocyte nuclei

Orthokeratosis

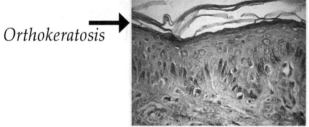

c. **Parakeratosis** - the retention of nuclei by keratinocytes in the stratum corneum

Column of parakera-tosis with surrounding ortho-keratosis

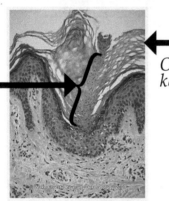

Ortho-keratosis

d. **Hypergranulosis** - increased granules in the keratinocytes of the stratum granulosum

Hypergranulosis

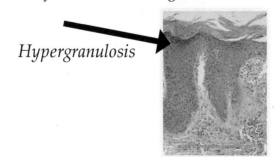

e. **Hypogranulosis** - decreased granules in the keratinocytes of the stratum granulosum

Hypogranulosis

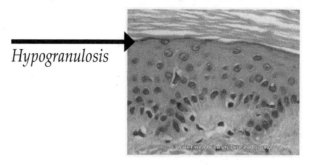

f. **Hyperplasia** - an increased number of cells
   i. *Psoriasiform* - regular acanthosis with elongated rete ridges of the same length

Psoriasiform hyperplasia

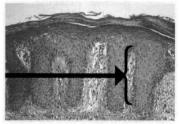

   ii. *Irregular* - acanthosis with rete ridges of differing lengths, often pointed

Irregular hyperplasia with pointed rete ridges

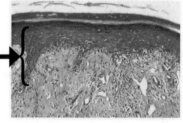

   iii. *Papillated* - thickening of the epidermis with nipple-like elevations

Papillated hyperplasia

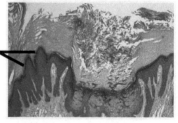

   iv. *Pseudocarcinomatous* - extreme, irregular thickening of the epidermis with increased mitoses, squamous eddies, or keratin pearls which may mimic squamous cell carcinoma

Keratin pearl

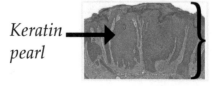

Irregular epidermal hyperplasia

1. Squamous eddy - concentric, whorled groups of keratinocytes with increased keratinization towards the center

Squamous eddy

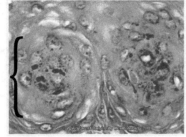

2. *Horn (or keratin) pearl* - a squamous eddy with more abrupt and complete keratinization

Keratin pearls

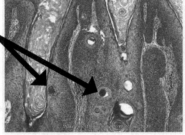

g. **Acanthosis** - diffuse epidermal hyperplasia, especially of the stratum spinosum

Acanthosis

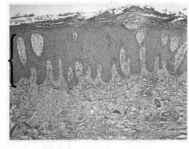

h. **Atrophy** - decreased thickness of a tissue or layer

Epidermal atrophy with loss of rete ridges and dermal papilla pattern

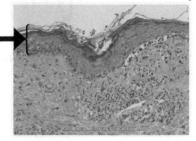

i. **Spongiosis** - intercellular edema expands the space between keratinocytes and can cause the cells to become elongated or stretched

Spongiosis and formation of intraepidermal vesicles

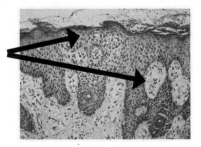

j. **Ballooning** - intracellular edema that eventually causes loss of attachment to adjacent cells (secondary acantholysis), generally due to viral particles

Ballooning degeneration of epidermal cells

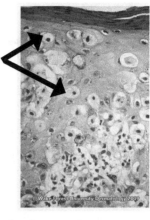

k. **Acantholysis** - the loss of cohesion between keratinocytes due to dissolution of intercellular connections (desmosomes) (see **Dyskeratosis** photo)

l. **Spongiform pustule** - collections of neutrophils in the spinous layer

Spongiform pustules

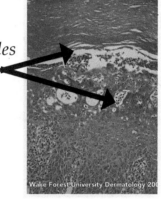

m. **Dyskeratosis** - abnormal or premature cornification of keratinocytes

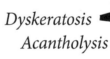

Dyskeratosis
Acantholysis

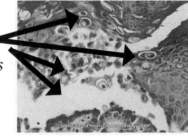

n. **Necrosis** - cell death with subsequent degeneration

Necrosis

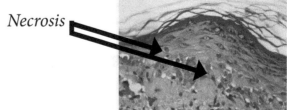

o. **Vacuolar alteration** - intracellular or extracellular clear space that causes damaged keratinocytes to appear vacuolated

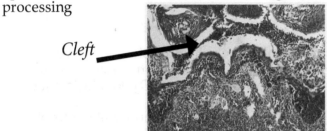

Vacuolar alteration

p. **Clefts** - an empty space, which may contain fluid, lipid, or other substances that is lost during tissue processing

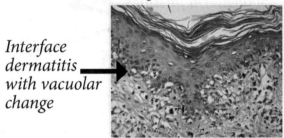

Cleft

q. **Interface dermatitis** - liquefactive degeneration of the basal cell layer at the interface between the epidermis and dermis with sparse inflammation

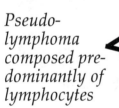

Interface dermatitis with vacuolar change

DERMAL

a. **Monomorphous infiltrate** - abnormal presence of inflammatory cells of one cell type

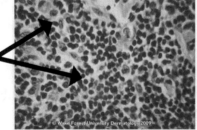

Pseudo-lymphoma composed predominantly of lymphocytes

b. **Mixed infiltrate** - abnormal presence of inflammatory cells of multiple cell types

Mixed infiltrate of lymphocytes, histiocytes, and eosinophils in urticarial pemphigoid

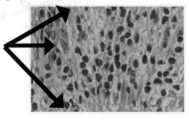

c. **Lymphohistiocytic infiltrate** - a collection of lymphocytes and histiocytes

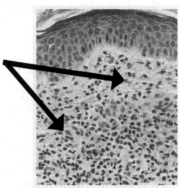

Mixed infiltrate of lymphocytes and histiocytes in pigmented purpuric dermatosis

d. **Lichenoid infiltrate** - a band-like configuration of inflammatory cells arranged parallel to the dermis

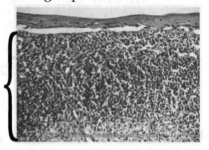

Band-like, lichenoid infiltrate seen in lichenoid drug reaction

e. **Nodular infiltrate** - dense discrete aggregations of inflammatory or tumor cells

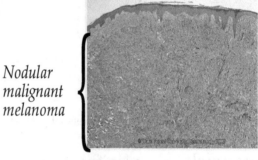

Nodular malignant melanoma

f. **Leukocytoclastic infiltrate** - collection of abnormal neutrophils characterized by chromatin fragmentation, nuclear dust, and necrotic debris

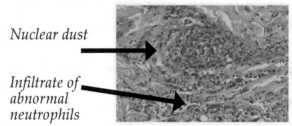

Nuclear dust

Infiltrate of abnormal neutrophils

g. **Diffuse infiltrate** - an infiltrate of inflammatory or tumor cells distributed in a nonlocalized fashion

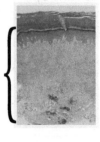

Diffuse infiltrate in superficial and deep dermis

CONNECTIVE TISSUE

a. **Collagen degeneration** - disorganized, fragmented mass of collagen (as opposed to the tightly packed, strictly aligned filaments normally seen)

Collagen degeneration alternating with areas of perivascular infiltrate

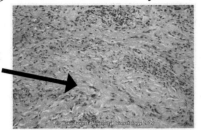

b. **Hyalinization of collagen** - relatively hypocellular, eosinophilic appearance of collagen

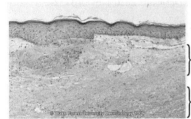

Hyalinized collagen with hypocellularity

More regular appearance of collagen compared to affected area above

c. **Fibrosis** - an increase in collagen associated with an increased number of fibroblasts

Increased collagen with an increased number of fibroblasts (at tip of lines)

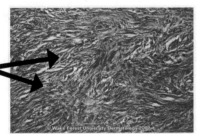

d. **Sclerosis** - an increase in collagen with either a normal or decreased number of fibroblasts

Thickened collagen throughout the dermis with decreased cellularity

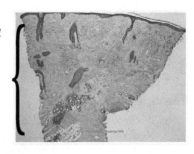

e. **Collagen in vertical streaks** - a vertical orientation of thick collagen bundles that occurs with chronic rubbing

Vertically streaked collagen within the papillary dermis

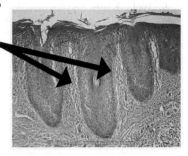

f. **Lamellated collagen** - layered, or plate-like arrangement of collagen

Whorls of layered collagen surrounding areas of increased melanocytes

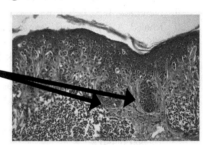

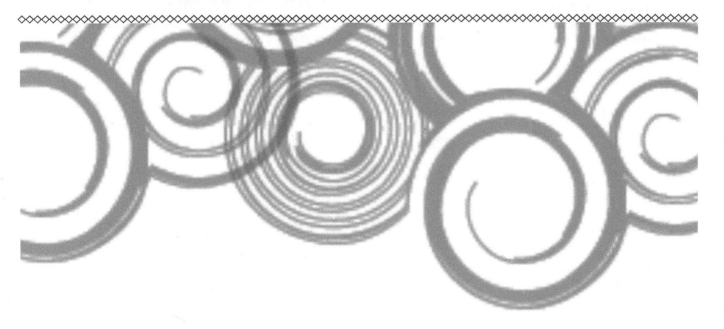

BIBLIOGRAPHY

1. Barnhill, Raymond L. *Dermatopathology*. New York: McGraw-Hill Medical, 2010. 193-94.
2. Elder, D., ed. *Lever's Histopathology of the Skin*. 8th ed. Philadelphia, PA: Lippincott-Raven Publishers, 1997:153.
3. Rapini, Ronald P. *Practical Dermatopathology*. Philadelphia: Elsevier Mosby, 2005, 53.
4. Ackerman, A. Bernard. *Histologic Diagnosis of Inflammatory Skin Diseases: A Method by Pattern Analysis*. Philadelphia: Lea & Febiger, 1978, 175–78.
5. Bolognia, Jean, Joseph L. Jorizzo, and Ronald P. Rapini. *Dermatology*. St. Louis, MO: Mosby/Elsevier, 2008. 326+.
6. Wolff, Klaus, Richard Allen Johnson, and Thomas B. Fitzpatrick. *Fitzpatrick's Color Atlas and Synopsis of Clinical Dermatology*. New York: McGraw-Hill, Medical Pub. Division, 2009. 144–45.
7. Burns, Tony, Stephen Breathnach, Neil Cox, and Christopher Griffiths. *Rook's Textbook of Dermatology, 7th ed*. Malden, MA. Blackwell Science 2004.
8. Kane, Kay S., Jennifer Bissonette, Howard P. Baden, Richard. A. Johnson, and Alexander Stratigos. *Color Atlas & Synopsis of Pediatric Dermatology*. New York: McGraw-Hill Professional, 2001.
9. Wolff, Klaus, and Richard A. Johnson. *Fitzpatrick's Dermatology in General Medicine, 7th ed*. New York: McGraw-Hill, 2008.
10. Ashton. R. and B. Leppard. *Differential Diagnosis in Dermatology*, 3rd ed. Oxon: Radcliffe Publishing Ltd, 2005.
11. Weedon, D. *Skin Pathology*. 2nd Ed. London: Churchill Livingstone. 2002:245–6.
12. Hu, Stephanie W., and Michael Bigby. *Pityriasis Versicolor: A Systematic Review of Interventions*. Arch Dermatol. 2010;146(10):1132–1140.
13. Sugar, Alan M. "Mucormycosis". In Fauci, A.S., Braunwald, E., Kasper, D.L., Hauser, S.L., Longo, D.L., Jameson, J.L., and Loscalzo, J.: *Harrison's Principles of Internal Medicine, 17e*. New York: McGrawHill 2008.
14. Krasteva, M., Kehren, J., Sayag, M., Ducluzeau, M.T., Dupuis, M., Kanitakis, J., et al. Contact dermatitis II. Clinical aspects and diagnosis. *Eur J Dermatol*. 1999 Mar;9(2):144–59.
15. Weitzman, I. and A.A. Padhye. Dermatophytes: gross and microscopic. *Dermatol Clin*. 1996 Jan; 14(1):9–22.
16. Tyring, S.K. Reactive Erythemas: Erythema Annulare Centrifugum and Erythema Gyratum Repens. *Clin Dermatol* 1993;11:135–9.
17. Weedon, David. "Arthropod-Induced Diseases." *Weedon's Skin Pathology*. London: Churchill Livingstone, 2009. 652-62.
18. Korkij, W. and K. Soltani. Fixed drug eruption. A brief review. *Arch Dermatol* 1984;120:520–4.
19. Newman, L.S., C.S. Rose, and L.A. Maier. Sarcoidosis. *N Engl J Med* 1997;336:1224–34.
20. Khaled, A., M. Jones, R. Zermani, B. Fazaa, K. Baccouche, S. Ben Jilani, M.R. Kamoun, Granuloma faciale. *Pathologica* 2007, 99, (5), 306–8.
21. Mason, A.R., G.Y., Cortes, J. Cook, J.C. Maize, and B.H. Thiers. Cutaneous blastomycosis: A diagnostic challenge. *Int J Dermatol*. 2008; 47: 824–830.
22. DiCaudo, D.J. Coccidioidomycosis: A review and update. *J Am Acad Dermatol*. 2006; 55(6): 929–42.
23. Epstein, J.H., D.L. Tuffanelli, and W.L. Epstein. Cutaneous changes in the porphyrias. A microscopic study. *Arch Dermatol*. May 1973;107(5):689–98.
24. Yancey, K.B. and C.A. Egan. Pemphigoid: Clinical, histologic, immunopathologic, and therapeutic considerations. *JAMA*. 2000 Jul 19;284(3):350-6.
25. Nikolas, M.E., P.K. Krause, L.E. Gibson, et al. Dermatitis herpetiformis. *Int J Dermatol*. 2003, 42:588–600.
26. Bertolino, A. and I. Freedberg, "Hair: Andro-Genetic Alopecia." *Dermatology in General Medicine, Fourth ed., Vol. 1*. New York: McGraw Hill, 1993. p. 679.
27. Odom, R., W. James, T. Berger, "Diseases of the Skin Appendages: Alopecia Areata." *Andrew's Diseases of the Skin: Clinical Dermatology, Ninth ed*. Philadelphia: W.B. Saunders Company, 2000. pp. 943–5.